Pediatric Nutrition

for Toddlers, School-aged Children, Adolescents, and Young Adults

A CLINICAL SUPPORT CHART

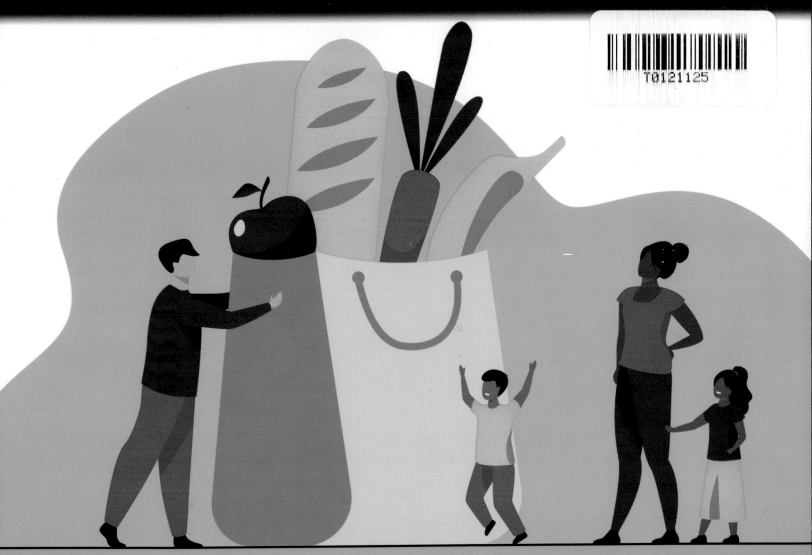

American Academy of Pediatrics

DEDICATED TO THE HEALTH OF ALL CHILDREN®

Thank you to the AAP Committee on Nutrition for their expert reviews.

American Academy of Pediatrics Publishing Staff
Mary Lou White, *Chief Product and Services Officer/SVP, Membership, Marketing, and Publishing*
Mark Grimes, *Vice President, Publishing*
Heather Babiar, MS, *Senior Editor, Professional/Clinical Publishing*
Theresa Wiener, *Production Manager, Clinical and Professional Publications*
Amanda Helmholz, *Medical Copy Editor*
Mary Louise Carr, MBA, *Marketing Manager, Clinical Publications*

Published by the American Academy of Pediatrics
345 Park Blvd
Itasca, IL 60143
Telephone: 630/626-6000
Facsimile: 847/434-8000
www.aap.org

The American Academy of Pediatrics is an organization of 67,000 primary care pediatricians, pediatric medical subspecialists, and pediatric surgical specialists dedicated to the health, safety, and well-being of all infants, children, adolescents, and young adults.

While every effort has been made to ensure the accuracy of this publication, the American Academy of Pediatrics does not guarantee that it is accurate, complete, or without error.

The recommendations in this publication do not indicate an exclusive course of treatment or serve as a standard of medical care. Variations, taking into account individual circumstances, may be appropriate.

Any websites, brand names, products, or manufacturers are mentioned for informational and identification purposes only and do not imply an endorsement by the American Academy of Pediatrics (AAP). The AAP is not responsible for the content of external resources. Information was current at the time of publication.

The publishers have made every effort to trace the copyright holders for borrowed materials. If they have inadvertently overlooked any, they will be pleased to make the necessary arrangements at the first opportunity.

This publication has been developed by the American Academy of Pediatrics. No commercial involvement of any kind has been solicited or accepted in the development of the content of this publication.

Every effort has been made to ensure that the drug selection and dosages set forth in this publication are in accordance with the current recommendations and practice at the time of publication. It is the responsibility of the health care professional to check the package insert of each drug for any change in indications or dosage and for added warnings and precautions.

Every effort is made to keep *Pediatric Nutrition for Toddlers, School-aged Children, Adolescents, and Young Adults: A Clinical Support Chart* consistent with the most recent advice and information available from the American Academy of Pediatrics.

Please visit www.aap.org/errata for an up-to-date list of any applicable errata for this publication.

Standard purchase price includes a license for one user. Licensing for additional users may be purchased.

Special discounts are available for bulk purchases of this publication. Email Special Sales at nationalaccounts@aap.org for more information.

First edition published 2024.
Printed in the United States of America
9-500/1023   1 2 3 4 5 6 7 8 9 10

MA1108
ISBN: 978-1-61002-683-3
eBook: 978-1-61002-684-0
Cover and publication design by LSD DESIGN LLC

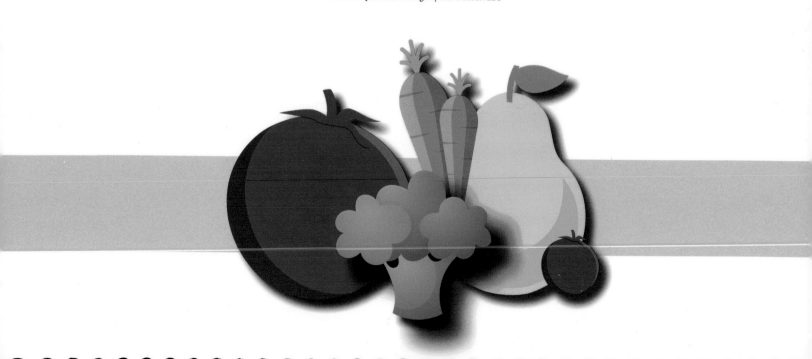

Contents

Equity, Diversity, and Inclusion Statement

The American Academy of Pediatrics is committed to principles of equity, diversity, and inclusion in its publishing program. Editorial boards, author selections, and author transitions (publication succession plans) are designed to include diverse voices that reflect society as a whole. Editor and author teams are encouraged to actively seek out diverse authors and reviewers at all stages of the editorial process. Publishing staff are committed to promoting equity, diversity, and inclusion in all aspects of publication writing, review, and production.

Please note that use of the terms *male* and *female* in this chart refer to biological/natal sex.

Medical Record Information

Significant information to gather from the medical record includes the following[a]:
- Reason for clinical visit or hospitalization
- Medical history
  - Diagnoses with emphasis on nutrition-related illnesses
  - Surgeries
- Current medications, vitamin and mineral supplements
- Laboratory data, medical tests, procedures
- Tanner stage
- Growth history
- Anthropometric measurements
  - Growth chart plots
  - z-Scores
- Prenatal and birth history (if <3 years old)

Interview Questions

Questions in the interview should gather information on the following topics:
- Social history
- Over-the-counter medications, vitamin and mineral supplements, and/or herbal supplements
- Oral-motor skills and swallow safety
- Dietary intake, including dietary supplements and any changes in intake (parenteral nutrition or enteral nutrition)
- Gastrointestinal symptoms
- Weight changes

Nutrition-Focused Physical Examination

Information to gather during the nutrition-focused physical examination includes the following:
- Anthropometric measurements (ie, height, with an alternative being knee height or arm span for individuals with impaired mobility; weight; weight gain velocity)
  - Visual assessment to verify that measurements documented in the medical record seem correct
- Additional measurements, such as mid-upper arm circumference
- Assessment of subcutaneous fat and muscle stores
- Assessment of the hair, eyes, oral cavity, skin, and nails for micronutrient deficiencies, as follows:

Nutrition-Focused Physical Examination Findings

Area	Normal Finding	Abnormal Finding	Related Nutritional Deficiencies
Hair	Smooth and symmetrically distributed	Poor quality	Zinc, essential fatty acid, biotin, protein-calorie
		Alopecia	Protein, zinc, biotin, essential fatty acid, selenium
Eyes	Bright, shiny, clear, pink moist membranes	Dull, dry membranes with Bitot spots	Vitamin A
		Burning, itching with photophobia	Riboflavin
Lips/mouth	Pink, free of lesions	Dry, swollen	Vitamin B_6, folate, riboflavin, niacin, vitamin B_{12}, iron
		Dry mucous membranes	Dehydration
		Dry mouth	Zinc
Tongue	Moist, pink with slightly rough texture	Magenta and edematous	Riboflavin, niacin, folate, vitamin B_6, vitamin B_{12}, iron
		Enlarged in congenital anomalies	May lead to feeding issues
		Candidiasis lesions or thrush	Vitamin C, iron

Area	Normal Finding	Abnormal Finding	Related Nutritional Deficiencies
Gums	Pink without lesions	Bleeding and inflamed	Vitamin C
Teeth	Normal eruption, which begins at age 4–12 months	Delayed eruption	Severe malnutrition
		Dental caries	Vitamin D
Skin	Uniform color without rashes, tears, or flaking	Pallor	Iron, folate, vitamin B_{12}
	Cool to the touch	Dry, scaly	Vitamin A, essential fatty acid
		Dermatitis	Essential fatty acid, zinc, niacin, riboflavin, tryptophan
Nails	Symmetrical and smooth	Transverse lines	Protein
		Flaky	Magnesium
		Poorly blanched	Vitamins A and C

Potential Elements of Nutritional Assessment for Children With Developmental Disabilities

- Medical history
- Nutrition-focused physical examination
- Complementary and integrative therapies
- Oral-motor concerns
- Nutritional/vitamin supplements
- Feeding skills
- Cognitive factors
- Social factors
- Anthropometric measurements
- Laboratory data
- Food intake pattern
- Bowel patterns
- Food insecurity
- Environmental factors
- Functional abilities

Nutrition-Related Medical Issues Frequently Seen in Children With Developmental Disabilities

Clinical Considerations	Potential Contributing Issues
Altered growth: onset; patterns, associated clinical issues	Short stature, underweight, overweight/obesity
Feeding: need for changes in formula, volume, rate, additives; recent changes in routines affecting feeding schedules (ie, home, school)	Feeding route: oral, enteral, parenteral, or combination of these
Gastrointestinal: recent or worsening symptoms	Constipation, diarrhea, dumping syndrome, dysmotility, gastroesophageal reflux, malrotation
Orthopedic: conditions creating chronic pain or anatomical restrictions that affect feedings	Dislocated hips, scoliosis, contractures, osteopenia
Medications, complementary and integrative medicine	Drug-nutrient interactions, medication side effects
Dysphagia: potential for changes with age	Oropharyngeal, esophageal
Effects on energy needs and caloric expenditure	Muscle tone (hypotonia/hypertonia), mobility status, medication side effects, underlying diagnosis, degree/level of physical therapy

[a] From Nutrition Therapy Department, Le Bonheur Children's Hospital, Memphis, TN; and Akron Children's Hospital, Akron, OH.
Derived from American Academy of Pediatrics Committee on Nutrition. *Pediatric Nutrition.* Kleinman RE, Greer FR, eds. 8th ed. American Academy of Pediatrics; 2020:1044, 1045; and Corkins KG, Teague EE. Pediatric nutrition assessment: anthropometrics to zinc. *Nutr Clin Pract.* 2016;32(1):40–51.

TAB 2

Biochemical Nutritional Values

Normal Values: Biochemical Measurement of Specific Nutritional Parameters

Test	Age	Normal Range Male	Normal Range Female
Protein, Blood			
Serum albumin, g/dL[a]	1–3 y	3.5–4.6	3.5–4.6
	4–6 y	3.5–5.2	3.5–5.2
	7–19 y	3.7–5.6	3.7–5.6
	20+ y	3.5–5.0	3.5–5.0
Retinol binding protein, mg/dL[b]		3.0–6.0	3.0–6.0
Blood urea nitrogen, mg/dL[a]	0–2 y	2.0–19.0	2.0–19.0
	3–12 y	5.0–17.0	5.0–17.0
	13–18 y	7.0–18.0	7.0–18.0
	19–20 y	8.0–21.0	8.0–21.0
	21+ y	9.0–20.0	7.0–17.0
Transferrin, mg/dL[a]		180–370	180–370
Prealbumin, mg/dL[a]	1–5 y	14.0–30.0	14.0–30.0
	6–9 y	15.0–33.0	15.0–33.0
	10–13 y	20.0–36.0	20.0–36.0
	14+ y	22.0–45.0	22.0–45.0
Protein, Urine			
Creatinine/height index		>0.9	>0.9
3-Methylhistidine, nmol/mg creatinine[a]	13 mo to 3 y	134–647	134–647
	4+ y	93–323	93–323
Creatinine (24-h), mg/d[b]	0–2 y	NA	NA
	3–8 y	140–700	140–700
	9–12 y	300–1,300	300–1,300
	13–17 y	500–2,300	400–1,600
	18–50 y	1,000–2,500	700–1,600
Hydroxyproline index		>2	>2
Vitamin A			
Serum or plasma retinol, μg/dL[b]	2 mo to 12 y	20–50	20–50
	13–17 y	26–70	26–70
	18+ y	30–120	30–120

Test	Age	Normal Range Male	Normal Range Female
Vitamin D			
25-OH-D$_3$, ng/mL[a]		>20	>20
1-25-OH-D$_3$, pg/mL[b]		15–75	15–75
Folic Acid			
Serum folate, ng/mL[a]	2–3 y	2.5–15.0	1.7–15.7
	4–6 y	0.5–13.0	2.7–14.1
	7–9 y	2.3–11.9	2.4–13.4
	10–12 y	1.5–10.8	1.0–10.2
	13–17 y	1.2–8.8	1.2–7.2
	18+ y	2.8–13.5	2.8–13.0
Red blood cell folate, ng/mL[b]		280–903	280–903
Vitamin K			
Prothrombin time, sec[a]	6+ mo	11.7–13.2	11.7–13.2
Vitamin E			
Serum or plasma α-tocopherol, mg/L[a]	2–12 y	5.5–9.0	5.5–9.0
	13+ y	5.5–18.0	5.5–18.0
Vitamin C			
Plasma vitamin C, mg/dL[b]		0.4–2.0	0.4–2.0
Vitamin B$_{12}$			
Serum vitamin B$_{12}$, pg/mL[a]	2–3 y	264–1,216	416–1,209
	4–6 y	245–1,078	313–1,407
	7–9 y	271–1,170	247–1,174
	10–12 y	183–1,088	197–1,019
	13–17 y	214–865	182–820
	18+ y	199–732	199–732

TAB 2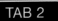

Biochemical Nutritional Values

Normal Values: Biochemical Measurement of Specific Nutritional Parameters (*continued*)

Test	Age	Normal Range Male	Normal Range Female
Iron			
Hematocrit, %[a]	2–5 y	34.0–40.0	34.0–40.0
	6–11 y	35.0–45.0	35.0–45.0
	12–17 y	37.0–49.0	36.0–46.0
	18+ y	41.0–52.0	36.0–46.0
Hemoglobin, g/dL[a]	2–5 y	11.5–13.5	11.5–13.5
	6–11 y	11.5–15.5	11.5–15.5
	12–17 y	13.0–16.0	12.0–16.0
	18+ y	13.5–17.0	12.0–16.0
Serum ferritin, ng/mL[b]	7–35 mo	12–57	12–60
	3–14 y	14–80	12–73
	15–19 y	20–155	12–90
	20–29 y	38–270	12–114
Serum iron, µg/dL[b]	1–10 y	50–120	50–120
	11+ y	50–170	30–160
Serum total iron binding capacity, µg/dL[b]	3 mo to 17 y	250–400	250–400
	18+ y	240–450	240–450
Serum transferrin saturation, %[b]		20–50	20–50
Serum transferrin, mg/dL[a]		180–370	180–370
Erythrocyte porphyrin (whole blood), µg/dL[b]		0–35	0–35
Zinc			
Serum zinc, µg/dL[a]	0–16 y	66–144	66–144
	17+ y	75–291	65–256

Test	Age	Normal Range Male	Normal Range Female
Phosphorus			
Serum phosphate, mg/dL[a]	1–3 y	3.8–6.5	3.8–6.5
	4–6 y	4.1–5.4	4.1–5.4
	7–11 y	3.7–5.6	3.7–5.6
	12–13 y	3.3–5.4	3.3–5.4
	14–15 y	2.9–5.4	2.9–5.4
	16–20 y	2.7–4.7	2.7–4.7
	21+ y	2.5–4.5	2.5–4.5
Calcium			
Serum total calcium, mg/dL[a]	1–3 y	8.7–9.8	8.7–9.8
	4–20 y	8.8–10.1	8.8–10.1
	21+ y	8.4–10.2	8.4–10.2
Serum ionized calcium, mmol/L[a]	2–4 y	1.21–1.37	1.21–1.37
	5–17 y	1.15–1.34	1.15–1.34
	18+ y	1.12–1.3	1.12–1.3
Magnesium			
Serum magnesium, mg/dL[a]	0–20 y	1.5–2.5	1.5–2.5
	21+ y	1.6–2.3	1.6–2.3
Copper			
Serum copper, µg/dL[b]	7 mo to 18 y	90–190	90–190
	19+ y	70–140	80–155
Selenium			
Serum selenium, µg/L[b]		23–190	23–190

NA indicates not available.

[a] Laboratory values from the clinical laboratories at Children's Hospital of Philadelphia.

[b] Laboratory values retrieved from ARUP laboratories (www.aruplab.com).

Adapted from American Academy of Pediatrics Committee on Nutrition. *Pediatric Nutrition.* Kleinman RE, Greer FR, eds. 8th ed. American Academy of Pediatrics; 2020:760–766.

TAB 3

Daily Nutritional Goals, Ages 2 and Older

Daily Nutritional Goals, Ages 2 and Older

Macronutrients, Minerals, and Vitamins	Source of Goal	M/F 2–3 y	F 4–8 y	F 9–13 y	F 14–18 y	F 19–30 y	M 4–8 y	M 9–13 y	M 14–18 y	M 19–30 y
Calorie Level Assessed		1,000	1,200	1,600	1,800	2,000	1,400	1,800	2,200	2,400
Macronutrients										
Protein (% kcal)	AMDR	5–20	10–30	10–30	10–30	10–35	10–30	10–30	10–30	10–35
Protein (g)	RDA	13	19	34	46	46	19	34	52	56
Carbohydrate (% kcal)	AMDR	45–65	45–65	45–65	45–65	45–65	45–65	45–65	45–65	45–65
Carbohydrate (g)	RDA	130	130	130	130	130	130	130	130	130
Fiber (g)	AI	19	25	26	26	25	25	31	38	38
Added Sugars (% kcal)	DGA	<10	<10	<10	<10	<10	<10	<10	<10	<10
Total lipid (% kcal)	AMDR	30–40	25–35	25–35	25–35	20–35	25–35	25–35	25–35	20–35
Saturated fatty acids (% kcal)	DGA	<10	<10	<10	<10	<10	<10	<10	<10	<10
18:2 linoleic acid (g)	AI	7	10	10	11	12	10	12	16	17
18:3 linoleic acid (g)	AI	0.7	0.9	1.0	1.1	1.1	0.9	1.2	1.6	1.6
Minerals										
Calcium (mg)	RDA	700	1,000	1,300	1,300	1,000	1,000	1,300	1,300	1,000
Iron (mg)	RDA	7	10	8	15	18	10	8	11	8
Magnesium (mg)	RDA	80	130	240	360	310	130	240	410	400
Phosphorus (mg)	RDA	460	500	1,250	1,250	700	500	1,250	1,250	700
Potassium (mg)	AI	2,000	2,300	2,300	2,300	2,600	2,300	2,500	3,000	3,400
Sodium (mg)	CDRR	1,200	1,500	1,800	2,300	2,300	1,500	1,800	2,300	2,300
Zinc (mg)	RDA	3	5	8	9	8	5	8	11	11

TAB 3

Daily Nutritional Goals, Ages 2 and Older

Daily Nutritional Goals, Ages 2 and Older (*continued*)

Macronutrients, Minerals, and Vitamins		M/F 2–3 y	F 4–8 y	F 9–13 y	F 14–18 y	F 19–30 y	M 4–8 y	M 9–13 y	M 14–18 y	M 19–30 y
Calorie Level Assessed	Source of Goal	1,000	1,200	1,600	1,800	2,000	1,400	1,800	2,200	2,400
Vitamins										
Vitamin A (mcg RAE[a])	RDA	300	400	600	700	700	400	600	900	900
Vitamin E (mg AT)	RDA	6	7	11	15	15	7	11	15	15
Vitamin D (IU)	RDA	600	600	600	600	600	600	600	600	600
Vitamin C (mg)	RDA	15	25	45	65	75	25	45	75	90
Thiamin (mg)	RDA	0.5	0.6	0.9	1.0	1.1	0.6	0.9	1.2	1.2
Riboflavin (mg)	RDA	0.5	0.6	0.9	1.0	1.1	0.6	0.9	1.3	1.3
Niacin (mg)	RDA	6	8	12	14	14	8	12	16	16
Vitamin B-6 (mg)	RDA	0.5	0.6	1.0	1.2	1.3	0.6	1.0	1.3	1.3
Vitamin B-12 (mcg)	RDA	0.9	1.2	1.8	2.4	2.4	1.2	1.8	2.4	2.4
Choline (mg)	AI	200	250	375	400	425	250	375	550	550
Vitamin K (mcg)	AI	30	55	60	75	90	55	60	75	120
Folate (mcg DFE)	RDA	150	200	300	400	400	200	300	400	400

AI indicates adequate intake; AMDR, acceptable macronutrient distribution range; AT, α-tocopherol; CDRR, chronic disease risk reduction level; DFE, dietary folate equivalent; DGA, *Dietary Guidelines for Americans, 2020–2025*; F, female; M, male; RAE, retinol activity equivalent; and RDA, recommended dietary allowance.

Sources: Institute of Medicine. *Dietary Reference Intakes: The Essential Guide to Nutrient Requirements.* National Academies Press; 2006; Institute of Medicine. *Dietary Reference Intakes for Calcium and Vitamin D.* National Academies Press; 2011; and National Academies of Sciences, Engineering, and Medicine. *Dietary Reference Intakes for Sodium and Potassium.* National Academies Press; 2019.

Adapted from US Department of Agriculture, US Department of Health and Human Services. *Dietary Guidelines for Americans, 2020–2025.* 9th ed. 2020. Accessed March 16, 2023. https://www.dietaryguidelines.gov/sites/default/files/2020-12/Dietary_Guidelines_for_Americans_2020-2025.pdf.

TAB 4

Caloric Needs per Day

Estimated Caloric Needs per Day, by Age, Sex, and Physical Activity Level, Ages 2 and Older

Age (y)	Male (calories)			Female (calories)		
	Sedentary[a]	Moderately Active[b]	Active[c]	Sedentary[a]	Moderately Active[b]	Active[c]
2	1,000	1,000	1,000	1,000	1,000	1,000
3	1,000	1,400	1,400	1,000	1,200	1,400
4	1,200	1,400	1,600	1,200	1,400	1,400
5	1,200	1,400	1,600	1,200	1,400	1,600
6	1,400	1,600	1,800	1,200	1,400	1,600
7	1,400	1,600	1,800	1,200	1,600	1,800
8	1,400	1,600	2,000	1,400	1,600	1,800
9	1,600	1,800	2,000	1,400	1,600	1,800
10	1,600	1,800	2,200	1,400	1,800	2,000
11	1,800	2,000	2,200	1,600	1,800	2,000
12	1,800	2,200	2,400	1,600	2,000	2,200
13	2,000	2,200	2,600	1,600	2,000	2,200
14	2,000	2,400	2,800	1,800	2,000	2,400
15	2,200	2,600	3,000	1,800	2,000	2,400
16	2,400	2,800	3,200	1,800	2,000	2,400
17	2,400	2,800	3,200	1,800	2,000	2,400
18	2,400	2,800	3,200	1,800	2,000	2,400
19–20	2,600	2,800	3,000	2,000	2,200	2,400
21–25	2,400	2,800	3,000	2,000	2,200	2,400

[a] *Sedentary* means a lifestyle that includes only the physical activity of independent living.

[b] *Moderately active* means a lifestyle that includes physical activity equivalent to walking approximately 1.5–3 miles per day at 3–4 miles per hour, in addition to the activities of independent living.

[c] *Active* means a lifestyle that includes physical activity equivalent to walking more than 3 miles per day at 3–4 miles per hour, in addition to the activities of independent living.

Source: Institute of Medicine. *Dietary Reference Intakes for Energy, Carbohydrate, Fiber, Fat, Fatty Acids, Cholesterol, Protein, and Amino Acids.* National Academies Press; 2005. Adapted from US Department of Agriculture, US Department of Health and Human Services. *Dietary Guidelines for Americans, 2020–2025.* 9th ed. 2020. Accessed March 16, 2023. https://www.dietaryguidelines.gov/sites/default/files/2020-12/Dietary_Guidelines_for_Americans_2020-2025.pdf.

TAB 5

Key Eating Recommendations and Serving Sizes

Key Eating Recommendations	
Nutrients	▸ Limit sodium, added sugars. ▸ Consume adequate potassium, fiber, vitamins D and E, calcium.
Foods	▸ Choose appropriate weaning foods. ▸ Avoid sugar-sweetened beverages. ▸ Avoid energy-dense, nutrient-poor snacks. ▸ Encourage vegetables, fruits, and whole grains. ▸ Encourage low-fat dairy or alternatives fortified with calcium and vitamin D.
Feeding	▸ Establish meal and snack routines, with limits. ▸ Provide small tastes of and repeated exposure to new foods. ▸ Model healthful eating.

Serving Sizes in Food Groups	
Food Group	**Serving Size**
Vegetable group	▸ 1 cup of raw, leafy vegetables ▸ ½ cup of other vegetables—cooked or raw ▸ 1 cup of vegetable juice
Fruit group	▸ 1 medium apple, banana, orange, or pear ▸ 1 cup of chopped, cooked, or canned fruit ▸ 1 cup of fruit juice
Milk, yogurt, and cheese group (milk group)	▸ 2 cups of fat-free milk or yogurt ▸ 1 ounce of natural cheese (eg, cheddar) ▸ 2 ounces of processed cheese (eg, American)
Meat, poultry, fish, dry beans, eggs, and nuts group (meat and beans group)	▸ 2–3 ounces of cooked lean meat, poultry, or fish ▸ ½ cup of cooked dry beans or ½ cup of tofu, either of which counts as 1 ounce of lean meat ▸ 2 ounces of soy burger or 1 egg, either of which counts as 1 ounce of lean meat ▸ 2 tablespoons of peanut butter or ⅓ cup of nuts, either of which counts as 1 ounce of meat
Bread, cereal, rice, and pasta group (grains group), whole grain and refined	▸ 1 slice of bread ▸ Approximately 1 cup of ready-to-eat cereal ▸ 1 cup of cooked cereal, rice, or pasta

Recommendations for Children With Type 1 Diabetes

▸ The mix of dietary carbohydrate, protein, and fat may be adjusted to meet the metabolic goals and individual preferences of the child with type 1 diabetes. There is insufficient evidence to support an "ideal" percentage of calories from carbohydrate, protein, and fat.

▸ Monitoring carbohydrate, whether by carbohydrate counting, choices, or experience-based estimation, remains a key strategy in achieving glycemic control. High-protein and high-fat foods and meals may require adjusted insulin dosing strategies.

▸ The use of the glycemic index and glycemic load may provide a modest additional benefit for glycemic control over that observed when total carbohydrate is considered alone.

▸ It is recommended that saturated fat intake be <7% of total calories.

▸ Reducing intake of trans-fatty acids lowers low-density lipoprotein and increases high-density lipoprotein concentrations; therefore, intake of trans-fatty acids should be minimized.

▸ Routine supplementation with antioxidants, such as vitamins E and C and beta carotene, is not advised because of lack of evidence of effectiveness and concerns related to long-term safety.

▸ Individualized meal planning should include optimization of food choices to meet recommended dietary allowance/Dietary Reference Intake for all micronutrients.

Adapted from American Academy of Pediatrics Committee on Nutrition. *Pediatric Nutrition.* Kleinman RE, Greer FR, eds. 8th ed. American Academy of Pediatrics; 2020:196, 856, 914.

TAB 6

Healthy Dietary Pattern for Ages 2–8 and 9–13

Healthy US-Style Dietary Pattern for Children Ages 2 Through 8, With Daily or Weekly Amounts From Food Groups, Subgroups, and Components

Calorie Level of Pattern[a]	1,000	1,200	1,400	1,600	1,800	2,000
Food Group or Subgroup	Daily Amount of Food From Each Group (Vegetable and protein foods subgroup amounts are per week.)					
Vegetables (cup eq/day)	1	1½	1½	2	2½	2½
	Vegetable Subgroups in Weekly Amounts					
Dark-green vegetables (cup eq/wk)	½	1	1	1½	1½	1½
Red and orange vegetables (cup eq/wk)	2½	3	3	4	5½	5½
Beans, peas, lentils (cup eq/wk)	½	½	½	1	1½	1½
Starchy vegetables (cup eq/wk)	2	3½	3½	4	5	5
Other vegetables (cup eq/wk)	1½	2½	2½	3½	4	4
Fruits (cup eq/day)	1	1	1½	1½	1½	2
Grains (ounce eq/day)	3	4	5	5	6	6
Whole grains (ounce eq/day)	1½	2	2½	3	3	3
Refined grains (ounce eq/day)	1½	2	2½	2	3	3
Dairy (cup eq/day)	2	2½	2½	2½	2½	2½
Protein foods (ounce eq/day)	2	3	4	5	5	5½
	Protein Foods Subgroups in Weekly Amounts					
Meats, poultry, eggs (ounce eq/wk)	10	14	19	23	23	26
Seafood (ounce eq/wk)[b]	2–3[c]	4	6	8	8	8
Nuts, seeds, soy products (ounce eq/wk)	2	2	3	4	4	5
Oils (grams/day)	15	17	17	22	22	24
Limit on calories for other uses (kcal/day)[d]	130	80	90	150	190	280
Limit on calories for other uses (%/day)	13%	7%	6%	9%	10%	14%

[a] Calorie level ranges: Ages 2 through 4, Females: 1,000–1,400 calories; Males: 1,000–1,600 calories. Ages 5 through 8, Females: 1,200–1,800 calories; Males: 1,200–2,000 calories. Energy levels are calculated based on reference height (median) and reference weight (healthy) corresponding with a healthy body mass index. Calorie needs vary based on many factors. The DRI Calculator for Healthcare Professionals, available at nal.usda.gov/human-nutrition-and-food-safety/dri-calculator, can be used to estimate calorie needs based on age, sex, height, weight, and activity level.

[b] The US Food and Drug Administration (FDA) and the US Environmental Protection Agency (EPA) provide joint advice regarding seafood consumption to limit methylmercury exposure for children. Depending on body weight, some children should choose seafood lowest in methylmercury or eat less seafood than the amounts in the Healthy US-Style Dietary Pattern. More information is available on the FDA and EPA websites at FDA.gov/fishadvice and EPA.gov/fishadvice.

[c] If consuming up to 2 ounces of seafood per week, children should only be fed cooked varieties from the "Best Choices" list in the FDA/EPA joint "Advice About Eating Fish," available at FDA.gov/fishadvice and EPA.gov/fishadvice. If consuming up to 3 ounces of seafood per week, children should only be fed cooked varieties from the "Best Choices" list that contain even lower methylmercury: flatfish (eg, flounder), salmon, tilapia, shrimp, catfish, crab, trout, haddock, oysters, sardines, squid, pollock, anchovies, crawfish, mullet, scallops, whiting, clams, shad, and Atlantic mackerel. If consuming up to 3 ounces of seafood per week, many commonly consumed varieties of seafood should be avoided because they cannot be consumed at 3 ounces per week by children without the potential of exceeding safe methylmercury limits; examples that should not be consumed include canned light tuna or white (albacore) tuna, cod, perch, black sea bass. For a complete list please see FDA.gov/fishadvice and EPA.gov/fishadvice.

[d] Foods are assumed to be in nutrient-dense forms; lean or low-fat; and prepared with minimal added sugars, refined starches, saturated fat, or sodium. If all food choices to meet food group recommendations are in nutrient-dense forms, a small number of calories remain within the overall limit of the pattern (ie, limit on calories for other uses). The number of calories depends on the total calorie level of the pattern and the amounts of food from each food group required to meet nutritional goals. Calories up to the specified limit can be used for added sugars and/or saturated fat, or to eat more than the recommended amount of food in a food group.

Note: The total dietary pattern should not exceed *Dietary Guidelines* limits for added sugars and saturated fat; be within the acceptable macronutrient distribution ranges for protein, carbohydrate, and total fats; and stay within calorie limits. Values are rounded.

From US Department of Agriculture, US Department of Health and Human Services. *Dietary Guidelines for Americans, 2020–2025.* 9th ed. 2020. Accessed March 17, 2023. https://www.dietaryguidelines.gov/sites/default/files/2020-12/Dietary_Guidelines_for_Americans_2020-2025.pdf.

TAB 6

Healthy Dietary Pattern for Ages 2–8 and 9–13

Children and Adolescents Ages 9 Through 13

In the late childhood and early adolescence stage, female children require about 1,400 to 2,200 calories per day and male children require about 1,600 to 2,600 calories per day.

Healthy US-Style Dietary Pattern for Children and Adolescents Ages 9 Through 13, With Daily or Weekly Amounts From Food Groups, Subgroups, and Components

Calorie Level of Pattern[a] Food Group or Subgroup	1,400	1,600	1,800	2,000	2,200	2,400	2,600
	Daily Amount of Food From Each Group (Vegetable and protein foods subgroup amounts are per week.)						
Vegetables (cup eq/day)	1½	2	2½	2½	3	3	3½
	Vegetable Subgroups in Weekly Amounts						
Dark-green vegetables (cup eq/wk)	1	1½	1½	1½	2	2	2½
Red and orange vegetables (cup eq/wk)	3	4	5½	5½	6	6	7
Beans, peas, lentils (cup eq/wk)	½	1	1½	1½	2	2	2½
Starchy vegetables (cup eq/wk)	3½	4	5	5	6	6	7
Other vegetables (cup eq/wk)	2½	3½	4	4	5	5	5½
Fruits (cup eq/day)	1½	1½	1½	2	2	2	2
Grains (ounce eq/day)	5	5	6	6	7	8	9
Whole grains (ounce eq/day)	2½	3	3	3	3½	4	4½
Refined grains (ounce eq/day)	2½	2	3	3	3½	4	4½
Dairy (cup eq/day)	3	3	3	3	3	3	3
Protein foods (ounce eq/day)	4	5	5	5½	6	6½	6½
	Protein Foods Subgroups in Weekly Amounts						
Meats, poultry, eggs (ounce eq/wk)	19	23	23	26	28	31	31
Seafood (ounce eq/wk)[b]	6	8	8	8	9	10	10
Nuts, seeds, soy products (ounce eq/wk)	3	4	4	5	5	5	5
Oils (grams/day)	17	22	24	27	29	31	34
Limit on calories for other uses (kcal/day)[c]	50	100	140	240	250	320	350
Limit on calories for other uses (%/day)	4%	6%	8%	12%	11%	13%	13%

[a] Calorie level ranges: Females: 1,400–2,200; Males: 1,600–2,600. Energy levels are calculated based on reference height (median) and reference weight (healthy) corresponding with a healthy body mass index. Calorie needs vary based on many factors. The DRI Calculator for Healthcare Professionals, available at nal.usda.gov/human-nutrition-and-food-safety/dri-calculator, can be used to estimate calorie needs based on age, sex, height, weight, and activity level.

[b] The US Food and Drug Administration (FDA) and the US Environmental Protection Agency (EPA) provide joint advice regarding seafood consumption to limit methylmercury exposure for children. Depending on body weight, some children should choose seafood lowest in methylmercury or eat less seafood than the amounts in the Healthy US-Style Dietary Pattern. More information is available on the FDA and EPA websites at FDA.gov/fishadvice and EPA.gov/fishadvice.

[c] All foods are assumed to be in nutrient-dense forms; lean or low-fat; and prepared with minimal added sugars, saturated fat, refined starches, or sodium. If all food choices to meet food group recommendations are in nutrient-dense forms, a small number of calories remain within the overall limit of the pattern (ie, limit on calories for other uses). The number of calories depends on the total calorie level of the pattern and the amounts of food from each food group required to meet nutritional goals. Calories up to the specified limit can be used for added sugars and/or saturated fat, or to eat more than the recommended amount of food in a food group.

Note: The total dietary pattern should not exceed *Dietary Guidelines* limits for added sugars and saturated fat; be within the acceptable macronutrient distribution ranges for protein, carbohydrate, and total fats; and stay within calorie limits. Values are rounded.

From US Department of Agriculture, US Department of Health and Human Services. *Dietary Guidelines for Americans, 2020–2025*. 9th ed. 2020. Accessed March 17, 2023. https://www.dietaryguidelines.gov/sites/default/files/2020-12/Dietary_Guidelines_for_Americans_2020-2025.pdf.

TAB 7

Healthy Dietary Pattern for Ages 14–18

Adolescents Ages 14 Through 18

Female adolescents require about 1,800 to 2,400 calories per day, and male adolescents require about 2,000 to 3,200 calories per day.

Healthy US-Style Dietary Pattern for Adolescents Ages 14 Through 18, With Daily or Weekly Amounts From Food Groups, Subgroups, and Components

Calorie Level of Pattern[a]	1,800	2,000	2,200	2,400	2,600	2,800	3,000	3,200
Food Group or Subgroup	Daily Amount of Food From Each Group (Vegetable and protein foods subgroup amounts are per week.)							
Vegetables (cup eq/day)	2½	2½	3	3	3½	3½	4	4
	Vegetable Subgroups in Weekly Amounts							
Dark-green vegetables (cup eq/wk)	1½	1½	2	2	2½	2½	2½	2½
Red and orange vegetables (cup eq/wk)	5½	5½	6	6	7	7	7½	7½
Beans, peas, lentils (cup eq/wk)	1½	1½	2	2	2½	2½	3	3
Starchy vegetables (cup eq/wk)	5	5	6	6	7	7	8	8
Other vegetables (cup eq/wk)	4	4	5	5	5½	5½	7	7
Fruits (cup eq/day)	1½	2	2	2	2	2½	2½	2½
Grains (ounce eq/day)	6	6	7	8	9	10	10	10
Whole grains (ounce eq/day)	3	3	3½	4	4½	5	5	5
Refined grains (ounce eq/day)	3	3	3½	4	4½	5	5	5
Dairy (cup eq/day)	3	3	3	3	3	3	3	3
Protein foods (ounce eq/day)	5	5½	6	6½	6½	7	7	7
	Protein Foods Subgroups in Weekly Amounts							
Meats, poultry, eggs (ounce eq/wk)	23	26	28	31	31	33	33	33
Seafood (ounce eq/wk)	8	8	9	10	10	10	10	10
Nuts, seeds, soy products (ounce eq/wk)	4	5	5	5	5	6	6	6
Oils (grams/day)	24	27	29	31	34	36	44	51
Limit on calories for other uses (kcal/day)[b]	140	240	250	320	350	370	440	580
Limit on calories for other uses (%/day)	8%	12%	11%	13%	13%	13%	15%	18%

[a] Calorie level ranges: Females: 1,800–2,400 calories; Males: 2,000–3,200 calories. Energy levels are calculated based on reference height (median) and reference weight (healthy) corresponding with a healthy body mass index. Calorie needs vary based on many factors. The DRI Calculator for Healthcare Professionals, available at nal.usda.gov/human-nutrition-and-food-safety/dri-calculator, can be used to estimate calorie needs based on age, sex, height, weight, activity level.

[b] All foods are assumed to be in nutrient-dense forms; lean or low-fat; and prepared with minimal added sugars, saturated fat, refined starches, or sodium. If all food choices to meet food group recommendations are in nutrient-dense forms, a small number of calories remain within the overall limit of the pattern (ie, limit on calories for other uses). The number of calories depends on the total calorie level of the pattern and the amounts of food from each food group required to meet nutritional goals. Calories up to the specified limit can be used for added sugars and/or saturated fat, or to eat more than the recommended amount of food in a food group.

Note: The total dietary pattern should not exceed *Dietary Guidelines* limits for added sugars and saturated fat; be within the acceptable macronutrient distribution ranges for protein, carbohydrate, and total fats; and stay within calorie limits. Values are rounded.

From US Department of Agriculture, US Department of Health and Human Services. *Dietary Guidelines for Americans, 2020–2025*. 9th ed. 2020. Accessed March 17, 2023. https://www.dietaryguidelines.gov/sites/default/files/2020-12/Dietary_Guidelines_for_Americans_2020-2025.pdf.

TAB 8

Additional Adolescent Nutrient-Specific Concerns

Daily Increments in Body Content of Minerals and Nitrogen During Adolescent Growth

Mineral	Sex	Average for 10–20 y, mg	Average at Peak of Growth Spurt, mg
Calcium	Male	210	400
	Female	110	240
Iron	Male	0.57	1.1
	Female	0.23	0.9
Nitrogen	Male	320	610
	Female	160	360
Zinc	Male	0.27	0.50
	Female	0.18	0.31
Magnesium	Male	4.4	8.4
	Female	2.3	5.0

Adapted from American Academy of Pediatrics Committee on Nutrition. *Pediatric Nutrition.* Kleinman RE, Greer FR, eds. 8th ed. American Academy of Pediatrics; 2020:230. Originally derived from Forbes GB. Nutritional requirements in adolescence. In: Suskind RM, ed. *Textbook of Pediatric Nutrition.* Raven Press; 1981:381–391.

Specific Nutrient Requirements and Concerns During Adolescence

Requirement/Concern	Clinician Guidance
Energy	The prevalence of overweight and obesity among adolescents aged 12–19 years remains alarmingly high, according to results from the current National Health and Nutrition Examination Survey. Obesity rates are higher in boys than in girls, and racial and ethnic disparities in rates persist.
Protein	Protein is required for growth, development, and maintenance of body tissues. The peak in protein intake correlates with the peak in energy intake, and during adolescence, protein needs, such as those for energy, correlate more closely with growth pattern than with chronological age. In the United States, mean protein intake is much greater than the recommended dietary allowances, so protein deficiency is not common but can occur in strict vegans, in chronic dieters, or in households with food insecurity.
Iron	The need for iron for male and female adolescents is increased during adolescence to sustain the rapidly enlarging muscle mass, expansion of blood volume, and increase in hemoglobin concentration; in female adolescents, it is needed to offset menstrual losses, and adolescent girls with menorrhagia are at increased risk of developing iron deficiency.
Zinc	Zinc is essential for growth and sexual maturation. Growth restriction and hypogonadism have been reported in male adolescents with zinc deficiency. Diets high in phytates can reduce the bioavailability of dietary zinc.
Vegan diets	Adolescents who consume no animal products may be vulnerable to deficiencies of several nutrients, particularly vitamins D and B_{12}, riboflavin, protein, calcium, iron, zinc, and, perhaps, other trace elements.
Dental caries	Although dental caries begin in early childhood, they are a highly prevalent nutrition-related problem of adolescence. Caries are associated with low fluoride intake in childhood and frequent consumption of foods containing carbohydrates. These include sugar-sweetened beverages, especially soda, which has been linked with poor oral health.
Conditioned deficiencies	A number of medications can interact with the absorption or metabolism of nutrients. Anticonvulsant drugs, especially phenytoin and phenobarbital, interfere with the metabolism of vitamin D and can lead to rickets and/or osteomalacia; therefore, supplementation with vitamin D may be desirable. Isoniazid interferes with pyridoxine metabolism. Oral contraceptives increase serum lipid concentrations, an effect that may have some clinical significance.
Chronic disease	Adolescents with chronic diseases such as inflammatory bowel disease, celiac disease, diabetes mellitus, juvenile idiopathic arthritis, or sickle cell disease may develop nutritional deficiencies as a result of a combination of dietary limitations, increased metabolic requirements associated with chronic inflammation, and ongoing nutrient losses through the stools or urine. These chronic diseases can profoundly affect nutritional status.
Calcium and vitamin D	Adolescents who do not get 600 IU of vitamin D per day through foods should receive a supplement containing that amount. Calcium needs are 1,300 mg/day for children and adolescents 9–18 years of age and 1,000 mg/day for young adults 19 years of age and older.

Adapted from American Academy of Pediatrics Committee on Nutrition. *Pediatric Nutrition.* Kleinman RE, Greer FR, eds. 8th ed. American Academy of Pediatrics; 2020:231–232.

Determinants of Protein Requirements in Young Athletes

Protein contains the building blocks that are needed for
▶ Growth and development
▶ Synthesis and repair of muscle and other tissue
  – Injury
  – Microtrauma associated with exercise

Protein requirements in athletes vary and depend on
▶ Growth and development
  – Protein requirements increase during periods of rapid growth.
▶ Training status
  – Protein requirements increase during periods of increased training volume and intensity.
  – Protein requirements are higher in novice athletes.
▶ Energy availability
  – Protein requirements are higher during periods of decreased energy availability (ie, weight loss).
    • Increased protein intake appears to minimize muscle catabolism.

Protein Content of Some Common Foods and Supplements Used by Athletes

Food	Protein (g)
Meats/Eggs	
Hamburger (3 ounces, extra-lean)	24
Chicken, roasted (3 ounces)	21
Tuna (3 ounces, water-packed)	20
Egg (1 large)	6
Dairy	
Cottage cheese (½ cup, low-fat)	14
Yogurt (8 ounces)	12
Milk (8 ounces, whole or skim)	8
Nonfat dry milk (2 tablespoons)	3
Beans/Legumes	
Tofu (½ cup)	10
Peanut butter (2 tablespoons)	10
Lentils (½ cup, cooked)	9
Black beans (½ cup)	8
Hummus (2 tablespoons)	3
Grains	
Pasta (1 cup, cooked)	7
Bread (whole wheat, 2 slices)	5
Other	
Protein supplements (per serving)	20–35
Promax bar	20
Clif bar (peanut butter flavor)	12
Carnation-brand instant breakfast (with 8 ounces skim milk)	12
PowerBar	10
Ensure (8 ounces)	9

Carbohydrate Content of Sample Food and Products Commonly Ingested During Sports Activities

Food	Carbohydrate (g)
Apple, 1 medium	21
Banana, 1 medium	27
Clif Builders bar, 1 chocolate mint	30
Clif Kid Zbar, 1 chocolate brownie	23
Fig Newtons, 2-ounce single-serve packet	39
Fruit Roll-Ups, 1 strawberry roll	11
Kashi chewy granola bar, 1 chocolate/peanut butter	21
Kind bar, 1 fruit and nut	17
Luna bar, 1 lemon zest	27
Nature Valley bars, 2 oats and honey	29
Nutri-Grain bar, 1 strawberry	24
Orange, ½ large	11
PowerBar Performance bar, 1 peanut butter	44
Pretzels, 1 ounce (approximately 18 mini pretzels)	23
Raisins, 1½-ounce box	22
Trail mix, ¼ cup (Planters tropical fruit and nut)	17

Adapted from American Academy of Pediatrics Committee on Nutrition. *Pediatric Nutrition.* Kleinman RE, Greer FR, eds. 8th ed. American Academy of Pediatrics; 2020:326, 339.

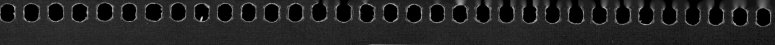

TAB 9

Nutrition for Young Athletes

Strategies for Weight Gain and Loss in Young Athletes

Strategies for Weight Gain in Young Athletes

GOAL: Maximize lean muscle gains and minimize fat gains

Potential rates of gains in lean muscle mass per week
▸ Girls and preadolescent boys: 0.25–0.75 pounds
▸ Postadolescent boys: 0.5–1.0 pounds

Training

High-intensity resistance training is a key aspect of making gains in lean mass.
▸ For muscle hypertrophy: 2–3 sets of 8–15 repetitions per set
▸ For strength/power gain: multiple sets of 4–6 repetitions per set

Appropriate rest
▸ Strength training for a given body part should be done on nonconsecutive days to allow muscle recovery in between high-intensity workouts.
▸ Adequate sleep should be obtained.

Nutrition

Calories
▸ Increase intake by 300–400 kcal/day over any increased expenditures.

Carbohydrates
▸ 1–4 g carbohydrates/kg body weight 1–4 hours before training provide fuel for a high-intensity workout and minimize muscle breakdown.

Protein
▸ Maintain 1.5–1.8 g/kg/day.
  – 0.3 g/kg within 2 hours after exercise and every 3–5 hours throughout the day

Fat—Consider increasing fat content of the diet if
▸ Difficulty gaining weight or ingesting adequate calories, after implementing the above recommendations
▸ No contraindications/other risk factors for a higher-fat diet

Practical Recommendations to Attain the Above

▸ Increase the frequency of meals/snacks.
▸ Do not skip breakfast.
▸ Aim to eat 5–9 times per day.
▸ Increase the size of meals/portions.
▸ Change the dietary composition to include nutrient-dense foods with higher caloric density.

Examples of ways to enhance calorie and/or protein content of foods in the diet
▸ Enrich full-fat milk with nonfat dry milk/instant breakfast.
▸ Reconstitute canned soup with evaporated milk instead of water.
▸ Choose cranberry, grape, or pineapple juice (in limited quantities), instead of orange or grapefruit juice.
▸ Add fruits and/or nuts to hot cereal, sandwich fillings, etc.
▸ Create sandwiches with thick-sliced, dense bread instead of white bread.

Weight Gain Supplements (ie, "Weight Gainers") Are Not Necessary

▸ US Food and Drug Administration regulation of supplements is much looser than for foods or drugs.
  – High rates of contamination/impure product

▸ Many provide between 500 and 2,000 kcal per serving.
  – If used as directed, will often result in excessive fat gains

▸ For young athletes, liquid food products (eg, Ensure, Carnation-brand instant breakfast) are reasonable options.
  – Regulated by the US Food and Drug Administration and widely available.
  – 2 servings per day often provide appropriate calories and protein to support lean tissue growth.

Strategies for Weight Loss in Young Athletes

GOAL: Maintenance of lean muscle mass while decreasing fat

Recommended rates of weight loss
▸ Growing athletes: up to 1 pound per week
▸ Skeletally mature athletes: up to 2 pounds per week

Training

▸ Monitor training quality and athletic performance during times of weight loss.
▸ Avoid detrimental effects of caloric/nutrient restriction.

Nutrition

Calories
▸ Decrease intake by 250–500 kcal/day; adolescents should not go below 1,600–1,800 kcal/day.
  – Reduce portion sizes and energy density of food.
    • Foods with low energy density include whole fruits/vegetables, whole grains, beans/legumes, low-fat dairy, and lean meats.

▸ Strategies consist of
  – Increase the proportion of vegetables in mixed dishes.
  – Use low-fat dairy/leaner meats.
  – Consume foods with high fiber and water content to increase satiety.
  – Eliminate sugar-sweetened beverages.

Carbohydrates
▸ Breakfast/a morning meal replenishes glycogen and provides fuel for activity.
▸ After a workout, carbohydrates replenish glycogen and provide fuel for the next workout.

Protein
▸ High intake of up to 2 g of protein/kg of body weight can help minimize loss of muscle mass during weight reduction.
▸ Spread protein intake throughout the day.
  – Is particularly important at breakfast and after working out
  – Provides a pool of amino acids for tissue maintenance and repair

Adapted from American Academy of Pediatrics Committee on Nutrition. *Pediatric Nutrition.* Kleinman RE, Greer FR, eds. 8th ed. American Academy of Pediatrics; 2020:346–347, 349.

TAB 10

Vegetarian and Vegan Diets

Healthy Vegetarian Dietary Pattern for Ages 2 and Older, With Daily or Weekly Amounts From Food Groups, Subgroups, and Components

Calorie Level of Pattern	1,000	1,200	1,400	1,600	1,800	2,000	2,200	2,400	2,600	2,800	3,000	3,200
Food Group or Subgroup	Daily Amount of Food From Each Group (Vegetable and protein foods subgroup amounts are per week.)											
Vegetables (cup eq/day)	1	1½	1½	2	2½	2½	3	3	3½	3½	4	4
	Vegetable Subgroups in Weekly Amounts											
Dark-green vegetables (cup eq/wk)	½	1	1	1½	1½	1½	2	2	2½	2½	2½	2½
Red and orange vegetables (cup eq/wk)	2½	3	3	4	5½	5½	6	6	7	7	7½	7½
Beans, peas, lentils (cup eq/wk)[a]	½	½	½	1	1½	1½	2	2	2½	2½	3	3
Starchy vegetables (cup eq/wk)	2	3½	3½	4	5	5	6	6	7	7	8	8
Other vegetables (cup eq/wk)	1½	2½	2½	3½	4	4	5	5	5½	5½	7	7
Fruits (cup eq/day)	1	1	1½	1½	1½	2	2	2	2	2½	2½	2½
Grains (ounce eq/day)	3	4	5	5½	6½	6½	7½	8½	9½	10½	10½	10½
Whole grains (ounce eq/day)	1½	2	2½	3	3½	3½	4	4½	5	5½	5½	5½
Refined grains (ounce eq/day)	1½	2	2½	2½	3	3	3½	4	4½	5	5	5
Dairy (cup eq/day)	2	2½	2½	3	3	3	3	3	3	3	3	3
Protein foods (ounce eq/day)	1	1½	2	2½	3	3½	3½	4	4½	5	5½	6
	Protein Foods Subgroups in Weekly Amounts											
Eggs (ounce eq/wk)	2	3	3	3	3	3	3	3	3	4	4	4
Beans, peas, lentils (cup eq/wk)[a]	1	2	4	4	6	6	6	8	9	10	11	12
Soy products (ounce eq/wk)	2	3	4	6	6	8	8	9	10	11	12	13
Nuts, seeds (ounce eq/wk)	2	2	3	5	6	7	7	8	9	10	12	13
Oils (grams/day)	15	17	17	22	24	27	29	31	34	36	44	51
Limit on calories for other uses (kcal/day)	170	140	160	150	150	250	290	350	350	350	390	500
Limit on calories for other uses (%/day)	17%	12%	11%	9%	8%	13%	13%	15%	13%	13%	13%	16%

[a] About half of beans, peas, lentils are shown as vegetables, in cup equivalents, and half as protein foods, in ounce equivalents. Beans, peas, lentils in the patterns, in cup equivalents, is the amount in the vegetable group plus the amount in protein foods group (in ounce equivalents) divided by 4.

Note: The total dietary pattern should not exceed *Dietary Guidelines* limits for added sugars, saturated fat, and alcohol; be within the acceptable macronutrient distribution ranges for protein, carbohydrate, and total fats; and stay within calorie limits. Values are rounded.

From US Department of Agriculture, US Department of Health and Human Services. *Dietary Guidelines for Americans, 2020–2025.* 9th ed. 2020. Accessed March 20, 2023. https://www.dietaryguidelines.gov/sites/default/files/2020-12/Dietary_Guidelines_for_Americans_2020-2025.pdf.

TAB 10

Vegetarian and Vegan Diets

Nutrients at Risk for Inadequate Intake in Vegetarian and Vegan Diets

Protein	Usually met with adequate energy intakes in a balanced vegetarian diet. Protein recommendations in vegans > 6 y are 20% more than for non-vegans because of decreased protein digestibility. Legumes and soy products can help ensure ingestion of balance of essential amino acids.	Supports tissue recovery and muscle building.
Essential fatty acids	Intake of long-chain omega-3 fatty acids (eicosapentaenoic acid [EPA] and docosahexaenoic acid [DHA]) is low in vegetarian diets. These can be endogenously synthesized from α-linolenic acid (ALA). Good ALA sources include variety of seeds and oils: flax, chia, canola, hemp, and walnut.	Inadequate intake can decrease calcium absorption.
Iron	Supports red cell production. Nonheme iron less absorption than heme iron (ie, meat-based). However, vitamin C/ascorbic acid and low iron levels (as often seen in vegetarians) can markedly enhance absorption.	Iron-deficiency anemia decreases athletic performance. Controversial impact of nonanemic iron deficiency on athletic performance. Some recommend routine monitoring of athletes, especially during periods of rapid growth.
Vitamin D	Supplements often needed (especially for indoor athletes and those living in northern climates).	Bone health, skeletal muscle function.
Zinc	Vegetarian diets generally lower than meat-based diets. Soaking and sprouting beans, grains and seeds can increase zinc bioavailability.	Impact of deficiency in athletes not known.
Calcium	Vegetable calcium sources are poorly absorbed. Tofu coagulated with calcium sulfate can be good source as well as fortified orange juice.	Bone health and muscle function.
Iodine	Variable amounts in dairy products. Sea vegetables and iodized salt are good sources.	Sweat losses can be significant. Role in athletic performance beyond impact on thyroid function is unknown.
Vitamin B$_{12}$	Not a component of plant-based foods. Milk and eggs contain vitamin B$_{12}$, but vegans need supplement or fortified foods.	Significant deficiency may cause anemia and decreased athletic performance. Mild deficiencies asymptomatic.

From American Academy of Pediatrics Committee on Nutrition. *Pediatric Nutrition.* Kleinman RE, Greer FR, eds. 8th ed. American Academy of Pediatrics; 2020:350–351.

The number of servings in each group is for minimum daily intakes. Choose more foods from any of the groups to meet energy needs.

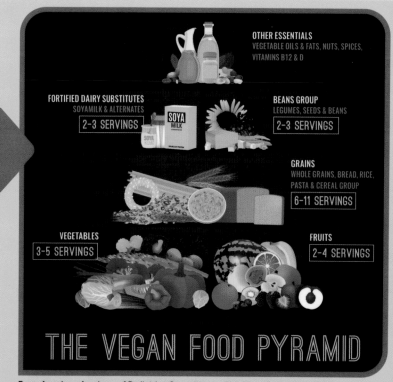

From American Academy of Pediatrics Committee on Nutrition. *Pediatric Nutrition.* Kleinman RE, Greer FR, eds. 8th ed. American Academy of Pediatrics; 2020:299.

Coronary artery disease and blood cholesterol levels are associated. The following risk factors have been identified for coronary heart disease: family history, increased serum total cholesterol level, reduced level of high-density lipoprotein cholesterol (HDL-C), increased level of low-density lipoprotein cholesterol (LDL-C), increased level of triglycerides, hypertension, cigarette smoking, diabetes mellitus, and lack of physical activity.

A diagnosis of hyperlipidemia can be confirmed after 2 separate serum lipid profiles are performed at least 2 weeks apart. Dietary therapy is the first mode of treatment in almost all instances, even if elevations are attributable to a genetic cause. Exceptions include extremely elevated LDL (generally ≥ 400 mg/dL) or triglyceride levels (generally ≥ 500 mg/dL) suggestive of a homozygous genetic lipid condition. A 3-day dietary record is helpful for suggesting changes; this record should be representative of the child's usual intake, including both weekdays and weekend days. Consultation with a registered dietitian is very helpful.

Interpretation of Cholesterol Levels for Children and Adolescents

Term	Total Cholesterol, mg/dL	LDL Cholesterol, mg/dL	HDL Cholesterol, mg/dL	Non–HDL Cholesterol, mg/dL	Triglycerides, mg/dL
Acceptable	<170	<110	>45	<120	<90
Borderline	170–199	110–129	40–44	120–144	90–129
High	≥200	≥130	(Low) < 40	≥145	≥130

To convert mg/dL to mmol/L, multiply by 0.02586 (cholesterol) or 0.0113 (triglycerides).

From American Academy of Pediatrics Committee on Nutrition. *Pediatric Nutrition.* Kleinman RE, Greer FR, eds. 8th ed. American Academy of Pediatrics; 2020:920. Originally from National Heart, Lung, and Blood Institute Expert Panel. Integrated guidelines for cardiovascular health and risk reduction in children and adolescents. *Pediatrics.* 2011;128(suppl 5):S213–S256.

FOR THE CHOLESTEROL CONTENT OF COMMON FOODS, SEE TAB 17.

nutrition guidance to reduce cholesterol

what foods to eat

➡ A variety of fruits and vegetables.

➡ Whole grain foods, such as whole grain bread, cereal, pasta, and brown rice. At least one-half of grains servings should be whole grains.

➡ Fat-free, 1%, and low-fat milk products.

➡ Poultry, without skin, and lean meats. When choosing to eat red meat and pork, select options labeled "loin" and "round." These cuts usually have the least amount of fat.

➡ Fatty fish such as salmon, trout, and sardines.

➡ Unsalted nuts, seeds, and legumes, including dried beans or peas.

➡ Nontropical vegetable oils, such as canola, corn, olive, and safflower oils.

what foods to limit

➡ Foods high in sodium

➡ Sweets and sugar-sweetened beverages

➡ Red meats and fatty meats that have not been trimmed

➡ Full-fat dairy products, such as whole milk, cream, ice cream, butter, and cheese

➡ Baked goods made with saturated and trans fats, such as donuts, cakes, and cookies

➡ Foods listed as containing "hydrogenated oils" in the ingredients list on the package

➡ Tropical oils, such as coconut, palm, and palm kernel oils

➡ Solid fats, such as shortening, stick margarine, and lard

➡ Fried foods

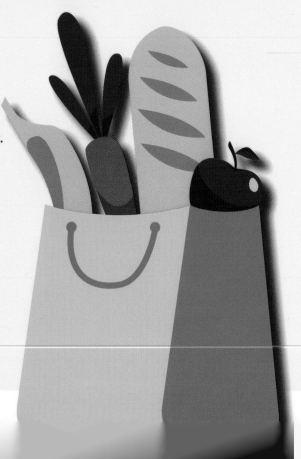

Derived from American Heart Association. *My Cholesterol Guide.* 2020. Accessed March 20, 2023. https://www.heart.org/cholesterol.

Screening for Hyperlipidemia

A nonfasting, non–HDL-C level can be used to evaluate a child's lipid status by 9 to 11 years of age and before the onset of puberty. This is determined by subtracting the HDL-C from the total cholesterol and has been found to be a useful risk indicator in adults and children, whether or not they are in a fasting state. If the non–HDL-C is ≥ 145 mg/dL, then a fasting lipid panel should be obtained. The following is an algorithm for screening and initiating therapy:

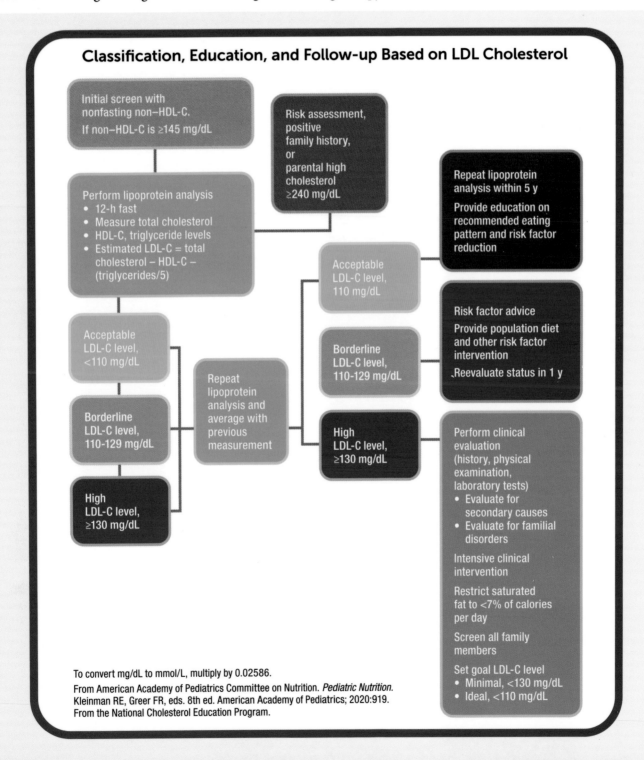

Classification, Education, and Follow-up Based on LDL Cholesterol

Initial screen with nonfasting non–HDL-C. If non–HDL-C is ≥145 mg/dL

Perform lipoprotein analysis
- 12-h fast
- Measure total cholesterol
- HDL-C, triglyceride levels
- Estimated LDL-C = total cholesterol – HDL-C – (triglycerides/5)

Risk assessment, positive family history, or parental high cholesterol ≥240 mg/dL

Acceptable LDL-C level, <110 mg/dL

Borderline LDL-C level, 110-129 mg/dL

High LDL-C level, ≥130 mg/dL

Repeat lipoprotein analysis and average with previous measurement

Acceptable LDL-C level, 110 mg/dL

Borderline LDL-C level, 110-129 mg/dL

High LDL-C level, ≥130 mg/dL

Repeat lipoprotein analysis within 5 y

Provide education on recommended eating pattern and risk factor reduction

Risk factor advice

Provide population diet and other risk factor intervention

Reevaluate status in 1 y

Perform clinical evaluation (history, physical examination, laboratory tests)
- Evaluate for secondary causes
- Evaluate for familial disorders

Intensive clinical intervention

Restrict saturated fat to <7% of calories per day

Screen all family members

Set goal LDL-C level
- Minimal, <130 mg/dL
- Ideal, <110 mg/dL

To convert mg/dL to mmol/L, multiply by 0.02586.
From American Academy of Pediatrics Committee on Nutrition. *Pediatric Nutrition*. Kleinman RE, Greer FR, eds. 8th ed. American Academy of Pediatrics; 2020:919. From the National Cholesterol Education Program.

(TAB 12)

Vitamin D

American Academy of Pediatrics Recommended Dietary Allowances for Vitamin D and Calcium

Age	Amount of Vitamin D per Day	Amount of Calcium per Day
1–3 years	600 IU	700 mg
4–8 years	600 IU	1,000 mg
9–18 years	600 IU	1,300 mg

Adapted from Porto A, Drake R. Cow's milk alternatives: parent FAQs. HealthyChildren.org. Updated June 2, 2022. Accessed March 20, 2023. https://www.healthychildren.org/English/healthy-living/nutrition/Pages/milk-allergy-foods-and-ingredients-to-avoid.aspx.

Vitamin D: Nutrient-Dense[a] Food and Beverage Sources, Amounts of Vitamin D and Energy per Standard Portion

Food[b,c]	Standard Portion[d]	Vitamin D (IU)	Calories
Protein Foods[e]			
Rainbow trout, freshwater	3 ounces	645	142
Salmon (various)	3 ounces	383–570	~115–175
Light tuna, canned	3 ounces	231	168
Herring	3 ounces	182	172
Sardines, canned	3 ounces	164	177
Tilapia	3 ounces	127	108
Flounder	3 ounces	118	73
Dairy and Fortified Soy Alternatives			
Soy beverage, unsweetened	1 cup	119	80
Milk, low fat (1%)	1 cup	117	102
Yogurt, plain, nonfat	8 ounces	116	137
Yogurt, plain, low fat	8 ounces	116	154
Milk, fat free (skim)	1 cup	115	83
Kefir, plain, low fat	1 cup	100	104
Cheese, American, low fat or fat free, fortified	1 1/2 ounces	85	104

TAB 12
Vitamin D

Vitamin D: Nutrient-Dense[a] Food and Beverage Sources, Amounts of Vitamin D and Energy per Standard Portion (*continued*)

Food[b,c]	Standard Portion[d]	Vitamin D (IU)	Calories
Vegetables			
Mushrooms, raw (various)	1 cup	114–1110	~15–20
Fruit			
Orange juice, 100%, fortified	1 cup	100	117
Other Sources			
Almond beverage (almond milk), unsweetened	1 cup	107	36
Rice beverage (rice milk), unsweetened	1 cup	101	113

[a] All foods listed are assumed to be in nutrient-dense forms; lean or low-fat and prepared with minimal added sugars, saturated fat, or sodium.

[b] Some fortified foods and beverages are included. Other fortified options may exist on the market, but not all fortified foods are nutrient-dense. For example, some foods with added sugars may be fortified and would not be examples in the lists provided here.

[c] Some foods or beverages are not appropriate for all ages, particularly young children for whom some foods could be a choking hazard.

[d] Portions listed are not recommended serving sizes.

[e] Seafood varieties include choices from the US Food and Drug Administration and US Environmental Protection Agency joint "Advice About Eating Fish," available at FDA.gov/fishadvice and EPA.gov/fishadvice from the "Best Choices" list. Varieties from the "Best Choices" list that contain even lower methylmercury include flatfish (eg, flounder), salmon, tilapia, shrimp, catfish, crab, trout, haddock, oysters, sardines, squid, pollock, anchovies, crawfish, mullet, scallops, whiting, clams, shad, and Atlantic mackerel.

Data Source: US Department of Agriculture, Agricultural Research Service. FoodData Central, 2019. fdc.nal.usda.gov.

From US Department of Agriculture, US Department of Health and Human Services. Food sources of vitamin D. Dietary Guidelines for Americans. Accessed March 20, 2023. https://www.dietaryguidelines.gov/food-sources-vitamin-d.

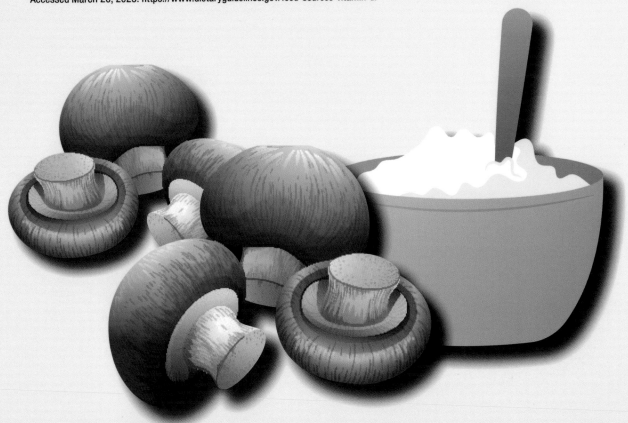

Iron: Nutrient-Dense[a] Food and Beverage Sources, Amounts of Iron and Energy per Standard Portion

Food[b,c]	Standard Portion[d]	Iron (mg)	Calories
Grains (Non-heme Sources)			
Ready-to-eat cereal, whole grain kernels, fortified	1/2 cup	16.2	209
Hot wheat cereal, fortified	1 cup	12.8	132
Ready-to-eat cereal, toasted oat, fortified	1 cup	9.0	111
Ready-to-eat cereal, bran flakes, fortified	3/4 cup	8.4	98
Protein Foods[e] (Heme Sources)			
Oyster	3 oysters	6.9	123
Mussels	3 ounces	5.7	146
Duck, breast	3 ounces	3.8	119
Turkey egg	1 egg	3.2	135
Bison	3 ounces	2.9	122
Duck egg	1 egg	2.7	130
Beef	3 ounces	2.5	173
Sardines, canned	3 ounces	2.5	177
Crab	3 ounces	2.5	98
Clams	3 ounces	2.4	126
Lamb	3 ounces	2.0	158
Turkey, leg	3 ounces	2.0	177
Shrimp	3 ounces	1.8	85
Organ meats (various)	3 ounces	1.8–19	~85–200
Game meats (various)	3 ounces	1.8–8.5	~115–180

Food[b,c]	Standard Portion[d]	Iron (mg)	Calories
Vegetables (Non-heme Sources)			
Spinach, cooked	1 cup	6.4	41
Artichokes, Jerusalem, cooked	1 cup	5.1	110
Hyacinth beans, cooked	1/2 cup	4.4	114
Soybeans, cooked	1/2 cup	4.4	148
Lima beans, cooked	1 cup	4.2	209
Swiss chard, cooked	1 cup	4.0	35
Chrysanthemum leaves, cooked	1 cup	3.7	20
Winged beans, cooked	1/2 cup	3.7	127
Stewed tomatoes, canned	1 cup	3.4	66
White beans, cooked	1/2 cup	3.3	125
Lentils, cooked	1/2 cup	3.3	115
Amaranth leaves, cooked	1 cup	3.0	28
Asparagus, raw	1 cup	2.9	27
Beets, cooked	1 cup	2.9	49
Moth beans, cooked	1/2 cup	2.8	104
Beet greens, cooked	1 cup	2.7	39
Jute, cooked	1 cup	2.7	32
Mushrooms, cooked	1 cup	2.7	44
Arrowroot, cooked	1 cup	2.7	78
Green peas, cooked	1 cup	2.5	134
Chickpeas (garbanzo beans), cooked	1/2 cup	2.4	135
Adzuki beans, cooked	1/2 cup	2.3	147
Pumpkin leaves, cooked	1 cup	2.3	15
Yard-long beans, cooked	1/2 cup	2.3	101
Mustard spinach, raw	1 cup	2.3	33

TAB 13

Iron-Dense Foods

Iron: Nutrient-Dense[a] Food and Beverage Sources, Amounts of Iron and Energy per Standard Portion (*continued*)

Food[b,c]	Standard Portion[d]	Iron (mg)	Calories
Vegetables (Non-heme Sources) (*continued*)			
Yellow beans, cooked	1/2 cup	2.2	128
Collard greens, cooked	1 cup	2.2	63
Navy beans, cooked	1/2 cup	2.2	128
Cowpeas, dried and cooked	1/2 cup	2.1	99
Poi (taro root)	1 cup	2.1	269
Peas in the pod, raw	1 cup	2.0	41
Kidney beans, cooked	1/2 cup	2.0	113
Pink beans, cooked	1/2 cup	1.9	126
Acorn squash, cooked	1 cup	1.9	115
Dandelion greens, cooked	1 cup	1.9	35
Great northern beans, cooked	1/2 cup	1.9	105
Leeks, cooked	1 cup	1.9	54
Potato, baked, with skin	1 medium	1.9	161
Cranberry (roman) beans, cooked	1/2 cup	1.9	121
Black beans, cooked	1/2 cup	1.8	114
Pinto beans, cooked	1/2 cup	1.8	123
Sweet potato, cooked	1 cup	1.8	190

Food[b,c]	Standard Portion[d]	Iron (mg)	Calories
Fruit (Non-heme) Sources			
Prune juice, 100%	1 cup	3.0	182
Protein Foods (Non-heme Sources)			
Sesame seeds	1/2 ounce	2.1	81
Cashews	1 ounce	1.9	157

[a] All foods listed are assumed to be in nutrient-dense forms; lean or low-fat and prepared with minimal added sugars, saturated fat, or sodium.

[b] Some fortified foods and beverages are included. Other fortified options may exist on the market, but not all fortified foods are nutrient-dense. For example, some foods with added sugars may be fortified and would not be examples in the lists provided here.

[c] Some foods or beverages are not appropriate for all ages, particularly young children for whom some foods could be a choking hazard.

[d] Portions listed are not recommended serving sizes.

[e] Seafood varieties include choices from the US Food and Drug Administration and US Environmental Protection Agency joint "Advice About Eating Fish," available at FDA.gov/fishadvice and EPA.gov/fishadvice from the "Best Choices" list. Varieties from the "Best Choices" list that contain even lower methylmercury include flatfish (eg, flounder), salmon, tilapia, shrimp, catfish, crab, trout, haddock, oysters, sardines, squid, pollock, anchovies, crawfish, mullet, scallops, whiting, clams, shad, and Atlantic mackerel.

Data Source: US Department of Agriculture, Agricultural Research Service. FoodData Central, 2019. fdc.nal.usda.gov.

Adapted from US Department of Agriculture, US Department of Health and Human Services. Food sources of iron. Dietary Guidelines for Americans. Accessed March 20, 2023. https://www.dietaryguidelines.gov/food-sources-iron.

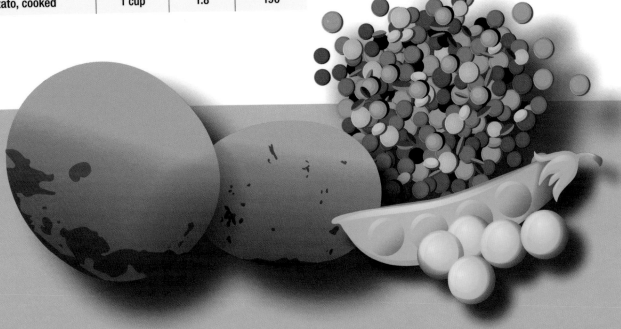

TAB 14

Calcium-Dense Foods

PLEASE SEE TAB 3 FOR RECOMMENDED DAILY CALCIUM INTAKE VALUES.

Calcium: Nutrient-Dense[a] Food and Beverage Sources, Amounts of Calcium and Energy per Standard Portion

Food[b,c]	Standard Portion[d]	Calcium (mg)	Calories
Dairy			
Yogurt, plain, nonfat	8 ounces	488	137
Yogurt, plain, low fat	8 ounces	448	154
Kefir, plain, low fat	1 cup	317	104
Milk, low fat (1%)	1 cup	305	102
Milk, fat free (skim)	1 cup	298	83
Buttermilk, low fat	1 cup	284	98
Yogurt, Greek, plain, low fat	8 ounces	261	166
Yogurt, Greek, plain, nonfat	8 ounces	250	134
Cheese, reduced, low, or fat free (various)	1 1/2 ounces	~115–485	~55–155
Vegetables			
Lamb's-quarters, cooked	1 cup	464	58
Nettles, cooked	1 cup	428	37
Mustard spinach, cooked	1 cup	284	29
Amaranth leaves, cooked	1 cup	276	28
Collard greens, cooked	1 cup	268	63
Spinach, cooked	1 cup	245	41
Nopales, cooked	1 cup	244	22
Taro root (dasheen or yautia), cooked	1 cup	204	60
Turnip greens, cooked	1 cup	197	29
Bok choy, cooked	1 cup	185	24
Jute, cooked	1 cup	184	32
Kale, cooked	1 cup	177	43
Mustard greens, cooked	1 cup	165	36
Beet greens, cooked	1 cup	164	39
Pak choi, cooked	1 cup	158	20
Dandelion greens, cooked	1 cup	147	35

TAB 14

Calcium-Dense Foods

Calcium: Nutrient-Dense[a] Food and Beverage Sources, Amounts of Calcium and Energy per Standard Portion (*continued*)

Food[b,c]	Standard Portion[d]	Calcium (mg)	Calories
Protein Foods[e]			
Tofu, raw, regular, prepared with calcium sulfate	1/2 cup	434	94
Sardines, canned	3 ounces	325	177
Salmon, canned, solids with bone	3 ounces	181	118
Tahini (sesame butter or paste)	1 tablespoon	154	94
Fruit			
Grapefruit juice, 100%, fortified	1 cup	350	94
Orange juice, 100%, fortified	1 cup	349	117
Other Sources			
Soy beverage (soy milk), unsweetened	1 cup	301	80
Yogurt, soy, plain	8 ounces	300	150
Almond beverage (almond milk), unsweetened	1 cup	442	36
Rice beverage (rice milk), unsweetened	1 cup	283	113

[a] All foods listed are assumed to be in nutrient-dense forms; lean or low-fat and prepared with minimal added sugars, saturated fat, or sodium.

[b] Some fortified foods and beverages are included. Other fortified options may exist on the market, but not all fortified foods are nutrient-dense. For example, some foods with added sugars may be fortified and would not be examples in the lists provided here.

[c] Some foods or beverages are not appropriate for all ages, particularly young children for whom some foods could be a choking hazard.

[d] Portions listed are not recommended serving sizes.

[e] Seafood varieties include choices from the US Food and Drug Administration and US Environmental Protection Agency joint "Advice About Eating Fish," available at FDA.gov/fishadvice and EPA.gov/fishadvice from the "Best Choices" list. Varieties from the "Best Choices" list that contain even lower methylmercury include flatfish (eg, flounder), salmon, tilapia, shrimp, catfish, crab, trout, haddock, oysters, sardines, squid, pollock, anchovies, crawfish, mullet, scallops, whiting, clams, shad, and Atlantic mackerel.

Data Source: US Department of Agriculture, Agricultural Research Service. FoodData Central, 2019. fdc.nal.usda.gov.

Adapted from US Department of Agriculture, US Department of Health and Human Services. Food sources of calcium. Dietary Guidelines for Americans. Accessed March 20, 2023. https://www.dietaryguidelines.gov/food-sources-calcium.

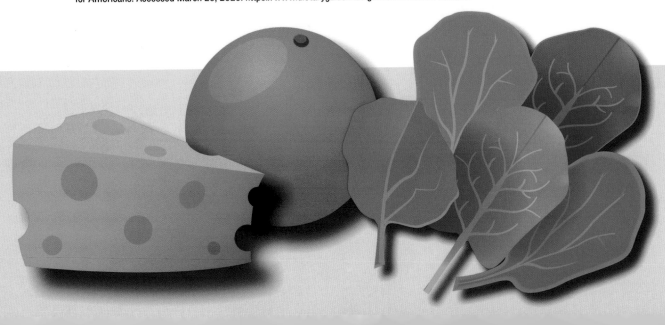

(TAB 15)

Fiber-Dense Foods

PLEASE SEE TAB 3 FOR RECOMMENDED DAILY FIBER INTAKE VALUES.

Dietary Fiber: Nutrient-Dense[a] Food and Beverage Sources, Amounts of Dietary Fiber and Energy per Standard Portion

Food[b,c]	Standard Portion[d]	Fiber (g)	Calories	Food[b,c]	Standard Portion[d]	Fiber (g)	Calories
Grains				**Vegetables** (*continued*)			
Ready-to-eat cereal, high fiber, unsweetened	1/2 cup	14.0	62	Nettles, cooked	1 cup	6.1	37
Ready-to-eat cereal, whole grain kernels	1/2 cup	7.5	209	Jicama, raw	1 cup	5.9	46
Ready-to-eat cereal, wheat, shredded	1 cup	6.2	172	Winter squash, cooked	1 cup	5.7	76
Popcorn	3 cups	5.8	169	Pigeon peas, cooked	1/2 cup	5.7	102
Ready-to-eat cereal, bran flakes	3/4 cup	5.5	98	Kidney beans, cooked	1/2 cup	5.7	113
Bulgur, cooked	1/2 cup	4.1	76	White beans, cooked	1/2 cup	5.7	125
Spelt, cooked	1/2 cup	3.8	123	Black-eyed peas, dried and cooked	1/2 cup	5.6	99
Teff, cooked	1/2 cup	3.6	128	Cowpeas, dried and cooked	1/2 cup	5.6	99
Barley, pearled, cooked	1/2 cup	3.0	97	Yam, cooked	1 cup	5.3	158
Ready-to-eat cereal, toasted oat	1 cup	3.0	111	Broccoli, cooked	1 cup	5.2	54
Oat bran	1/2 cup	2.9	44	Tree fern, cooked	1 cup	5.2	56
Crackers, whole wheat	1 ounce	2.9	122	Luffa gourd, cooked	1 cup	5.2	100
Chapati or roti, whole wheat	1 ounce	2.8	85	Soybeans, cooked	1/2 cup	5.2	148
Tortillas, whole wheat	1 ounce	2.8	88	Turnip greens, cooked	1 cup	5.0	29
Vegetables				Drumstick pods (moringa), cooked	1 cup	5.0	42
Artichoke, cooked	1 cup	9.6	89	Avocado	1/2 cup	5.0	120
Navy beans, cooked	1/2 cup	9.6	128	Cauliflower, cooked	1 cup	4.9	34
Small white beans, cooked	1/2 cup	9.3	127	Kohlrabi, raw	1 cup	4.9	36
Yellow beans, cooked	1/2 cup	9.2	128	Carrots, cooked	1 cup	4.8	54
Lima beans, cooked	1 cup	9.2	209	Collard greens, cooked	1 cup	4.8	63
Green peas, cooked	1 cup	8.8	134	Kale, cooked	1 cup	4.7	43
Adzuki beans, cooked	1/2 cup	8.4	147	Fava beans, cooked	1/2 cup	4.6	94
French beans, cooked	1/2 cup	8.3	114	Chayote (mirliton), cooked	1 cup	4.5	38
Split peas, cooked	1/2 cup	8.2	116	Snow peas, cooked	1 cup	4.5	67
Breadfruit, cooked	1 cup	8.0	170	Pink beans, cooked	1/2 cup	4.5	126
Lentils, cooked	1/2 cup	7.8	115	Spinach, cooked	1 cup	4.3	41
Lupini beans, cooked	1/2 cup	7.8	115	Escarole, cooked	1 cup	4.2	22
Mung beans, cooked	1/2 cup	7.7	106	Beet greens, cooked	1 cup	4.2	39
Black turtle beans, cooked	1/2 cup	7.7	120	Salsify, cooked	1 cup	4.2	92
Pinto beans, cooked	1/2 cup	7.7	123	Cabbage, savoy, cooked	1 cup	4.1	35
Cranberry (roman) beans, cooked	1/2 cup	7.6	121	Cabbage, red, cooked	1 cup	4.1	41
Black beans, cooked	1/2 cup	7.5	114	Wax beans, snap, cooked	1 cup	4.1	44
Fufu, cooked	1 cup	7.4	398	Edamame, cooked	1/2 cup	4.1	94
Pumpkin, canned	1 cup	7.1	83	Okra, cooked	1 cup	4.0	36
Taro root (dasheen or yautia), cooked	1 cup	6.7	187	Green beans, snap, cooked	1 cup	4.0	44
Brussels sprouts, cooked	1 cup	6.4	65	Hominy, canned	1 cup	4.0	115
Chickpeas (garbanzo beans), cooked	1/2 cup	6.3	135	Corn, cooked	1 cup	4.0	134
Sweet potato, cooked	1 cup	6.3	190	Potato, baked, with skin	1 medium	3.9	161
Great northern beans, cooked	1/2 cup	6.2	105	Lamb's-quarters, cooked	1 cup	3.8	58
Parsnips, cooked	1 cup	6.2	110	Lotus root, cooked	1 cup	3.8	108

TAB 15

Fiber-Dense Foods

Dietary Fiber: Nutrient-Dense[a] Food and Beverage Sources, Amounts of Dietary Fiber and Energy per Standard Portion (*continued*)

Food[b,c]	Standard Portion[d]	Fiber (g)	Calories
Vegetables (*continued*)			
Swiss chard, cooked	1 cup	3.7	35
Mustard spinach, cooked	1 cup	3.6	29
Carrots, raw	1 cup	3.6	52
Hearts of palm, canned	1 cup	3.5	41
Mushrooms, cooked	1 cup	3.4	44
Bamboo shoots, raw	1 cup	3.3	41
Yard-long beans, cooked	1/2 cup	3.3	101
Turnip, cooked	1 cup	3.1	34
Red bell pepper, raw	1 cup	3.1	39
Rutabaga, cooked	1 cup	3.1	51
Plantains, cooked	1 cup	3.1	215
Nopales, cooked	1 cup	3.0	22
Dandelion greens, cooked	1 cup	3.0	35
Cassava (yucca), cooked	1 cup	3.0	267
Asparagus, cooked	1 cup	2.9	32
Taro leaves, cooked	1 cup	2.9	35
Onions, cooked	1 cup	2.9	92
Cabbage, cooked	1 cup	2.8	34
Mustard greens, cooked	1 cup	2.8	36
Beets, cooked	1 cup	2.8	49
Celeriac, raw	1 cup	2.8	66
Fruit			
Sapote or sapodilla	1 cup	9.5	217
Durian	1 cup	9.2	357
Guava	1 cup	8.9	112
Nance	1 cup	8.4	82
Raspberries	1 cup	8.0	64
Loganberries	1 cup	7.8	81
Blackberries	1 cup	7.6	62
Soursop	1 cup	7.4	148
Boysenberries	1 cup	7.0	66
Gooseberries	1 cup	6.5	66
Pear, Asian	1 medium	6.5	75
Blueberries, wild	1 cup	6.2	80
Passion fruit	1/4 cup	6.1	57
Persimmon	1 fruit	6.0	118
Pear	1 medium	5.5	103
Kiwifruit	1 cup	5.4	110
Grapefruit	1 fruit	5.0	130
Apple, with skin	1 medium	4.8	104

Food[b,c]	Standard Portion[d]	Fiber (g)	Calories
Fruit (*continued*)			
Cherimoya	1 cup	4.8	120
Durian	1/2 cup	4.6	179
Star fruit	1 cup	3.7	41
Orange	1 medium	3.7	73
Figs, dried	1/4 cup	3.7	93
Blueberries	1 cup	3.6	84
Pomegranate seeds	1/2 cup	3.5	72
Mandarin orange	1 cup	3.5	103
Tangerine (tangelo)	1 cup	3.5	103
Pears, dried	1/4 cup	3.4	118
Peaches, dried	1/4 cup	3.3	96
Banana	1 medium	3.2	112
Apricots	1 cup	3.1	74
Prunes or dried plum	1/4 cup	3.1	105
Strawberries	1 cup	3.0	49
Dates	1/4 cup	3.0	104
Blueberries, dried	1/4 cup	3.0	127
Cherries	1 cup	2.9	87
Protein Foods			
Wocas, yellow pond lily seeds	1 ounce	5.4	102
Pumpkin seeds, whole	1 ounce	5.2	126
Coconut	1 ounce	4.6	187
Chia seeds	1 Tbsp	4.1	58
Almonds	1 ounce	3.5	164
Chestnuts	1 ounce	3.3	106
Sunflower seeds	1 ounce	3.1	165
Pine nuts	1 ounce	3.0	178
Pistachio nuts	1 ounce	2.9	162
Flaxseeds	1 Tbsp	2.8	55
Hazelnuts (filberts)	1 ounce	2.8	178

[a] All foods listed are assumed to be in nutrient-dense forms; lean or low-fat and prepared with minimal added sugars, saturated fat, or sodium.

[b] Some fortified foods and beverages are included. Other fortified options may exist on the market, but not all fortified foods are nutrient-dense. For example, some foods with added sugars may be fortified and would not be examples in the lists provided here.

[c] Some foods or beverages are not appropriate for all ages (eg, nuts, popcorn), particularly young children for whom some foods could be a choking hazard.

[d] Portions listed are not recommended serving sizes.

Data Source: US Department of Agriculture, Agricultural Research Service. FoodData Central, 2019. fdc.nal.usda.gov.

Adapted from US Department of Agriculture, US Department of Health and Human Services. Food sources of dietary fiber. Dietary Guidelines for Americans. Accessed March 20, 2023. https://www.dietaryguidelines.gov/food-sources-dietary-fiber.

TAB 16

Potassium-Dense Foods

PLEASE SEE TAB 3 FOR RECOMMENDED DAILY POTASSIUM INTAKE VALUES.

Potassium: Nutrient-Dense[a] Food and Beverage Sources, Amounts of Potassium and Energy per Standard Portion

Food[b,c]	Standard Portion[d]	Potassium (mg)	Calories
Vegetables			
Beet greens, cooked	1 cup	1,309	39
Fufu, cooked	1 cup	1,080	398
Lima beans, cooked	1 cup	969	209
Swiss chard, cooked	1 cup	961	35
Potato, baked, with skin	1 medium	926	161
Yam, cooked	1 cup	911	158
Acorn squash, cooked	1 cup	896	115
Amaranth leaves, cooked	1 cup	846	28
Spinach, cooked	1 cup	839	41
Breadfruit, cooked	1 cup	808	170
Bamboo shoots, raw	1 cup	805	41
Water chestnuts	1 cup	724	120
Carrot juice, 100%	1 cup	689	94
Taro leaves, cooked	1 cup	667	35
Plantains, cooked	1 cup	663	215
Taro root (dasheen or yautia), cooked	1 cup	639	187
Adzuki beans, cooked	1/2 cup	612	147
Cress, raw	2 cups	606	32
Butternut squash, cooked	1 cup	582	82
Parsnips, cooked	1 cup	572	110
Sweet potato, cooked	1 cup	572	190
Luffa gourd, cooked	1 cup	571	100
Chrysanthemum leaves, cooked	1 cup	569	20
Purslane, cooked	1 cup	561	21
Kohlrabi, cooked	1 cup	561	48
Broccoli rabe, cooked	1 cup	550	40
Drumstick pods (moringa), cooked	1 cup	539	42
Mushrooms, portabella, cooked	1 cup	529	35
Stewed tomatoes, canned	1 cup	528	66
Tomato juice, 100%	1 cup	527	41
Vegetable juice, 100%	1 cup	518	48
Mustard spinach, cooked	1 cup	513	29
Pumpkin, canned	1 cup	505	83
White beans, cooked	1/2 cup	502	125
Winter squash, cooked	1 cup	494	76
Artichoke, cooked	1 cup	480	89
Celeriac, raw	1 cup	468	66
Dandelion greens, cooked	1 cup	455	35
Cassava (yucca), cooked	1 cup	451	267
Burdock root, cooked	1 cup	450	110
Vegetables (continued)			
Bok choy, cooked	1 cup	445	24
Soybeans, cooked	1/2 cup	443	148
Lotus root, cooked	1 cup	440	108
Poi (taro root)	1 cup	439	269
Pink beans, cooked	1/2 cup	430	126
Small white beans, cooked	1/2 cup	415	127
Carrots, raw	1 cup	410	52
Black turtle beans, cooked	1/2 cup	401	120
Snow peas, cooked	1 cup	384	67
Corn, cooked	1 cup	384	134
Salsify, cooked	1 cup	382	92
Pinto beans, cooked	1/2 cup	373	123
Escarole, cooked	1 cup	368	22
Rutabaga, cooked	1 cup	367	51
Lentils, cooked	1/2 cup	366	115
Avocado	1/2 cup	364	120
Fennel bulb, raw	1 cup	360	27
Onions, cooked	1 cup	359	92
Kidney beans, cooked	1/2 cup	359	113
Split peas, cooked	1/2 cup	355	116
Navy beans, cooked	1/2 cup	354	128
Great northern beans, cooked	1/2 cup	346	105
Cowpeas, dried and cooked	1/2 cup	345	80
Cranberry (roman) beans, cooked	1/2 cup	343	121
Edamame, cooked	1/2 cup	338	94
French beans, cooked	1/2 cup	328	114
Hyacinth beans, cooked	1/2 cup	327	114
Pigeon peas, cooked	1/2 cup	323	102
Cauliflower, raw	1 cup	320	27
Red bell pepper, raw	1 cup	314	39
Black beans, cooked	1/2 cup	306	114
Nettles, cooked	1 cup	297	37
Summer squash, cooked	1 cup	296	18
Turnip greens, cooked	1 cup	292	29
Nopales, cooked	1 cup	291	22
Yellow beans, cooked	1/2 cup	288	128
Fava beans, cooked	1/2 cup	228	94
Collard greens, cooked	1 cup	222	63

TAB 16

Potassium-Dense Foods

Potassium: Nutrient-Dense[a] Food and Beverage Sources, Amounts of Potassium and Energy per Standard Portion (*continued*)

Food[b,c]	Standard Portion[d]	Potassium (mg)	Calories
Fruit			
Durian	1 cup	1,059	357
Sapote or sapodilla	1 cup	794	217
Jackfruit	1 cup	739	157
Prune juice, 100%	1 cup	707	182
Guava	1 cup	688	112
Passion-fruit juice, 100%	1 cup	687	126
Soursop	1 cup	626	148
Kiwifruit	1 cup	562	110
Pomegranate juice, 100%	1 cup	533	134
Orange juice, 100%	1 cup	496	112
Melon, cantaloupe	1 cup	473	60
Cherimoya	1 cup	459	120
Banana	1 medium	451	112
Tangerine juice, 100%	1 cup	440	106
Grapefruit	1 fruit	415	130
Pummelo	1 cup	410	72
Apricots	1 cup	401	74
Peaches, dried	1/4 cup	399	96
Loquats	1 cup	396	70
Melon, honeydew	1 cup	388	61
Apricots, dried	1/4 cup	378	78
Grapefruit juice, 100%	1 cup	362	95
Lychee	1 cup	325	125
Pineapple juice, 100%	1 cup	325	132
Mandarin orange	1 cup	324	103
Tangerine (tangelo)	1 cup	324	103
Prunes or dried plum	1/4 cup	319	105
Melon, casaba	1 cup	309	48
Raisins	1/4 cup	307	123
Cherries	1 cup	306	87
Gooseberries	1 cup	297	66
Peach	1 cup	293	60
Dairy and Fortified Soy Alternatives			
Yogurt, plain, nonfat	8 ounces	625	137
Yogurt, plain, low fat	8 ounces	573	154
Kefir, plain, low fat	1 cup	399	104
Milk, fat free (skim)	1 cup	382	83
Buttermilk, low fat	1 cup	370	98
Milk, low fat (1%)	1 cup	366	102
Yogurt, Greek, plain, nonfat	8 ounces	320	134
Yogurt, Greek, plain, low fat	8 ounces	320	166
Soy beverage, unsweetened	1 cup	292	80

Food[b,c]	Standard Portion[d]	Potassium (mg)	Calories
Protein Foods[e]			
Clams	3 ounces	534	126
Skipjack tuna	3 ounces	444	112
Shad	3 ounces	418	214
Mullet	3 ounces	389	128
Pollock	3 ounces	388	100
Rainbow trout, freshwater	3 ounces	383	142
Whiting	3 ounces	368	99
Herring	3 ounces	356	172
Goat	3 ounces	344	122
Tempeh	1/2 cup	342	160
Atlantic mackerel	3 ounces	341	223
Sardines, canned	3 ounces	338	177
Tilapia	3 ounces	323	108
Cod	3 ounces	316	71
Smelt	3 ounces	316	105
Catfish	3 ounces	311	122
Bison	3 ounces	307	122
Pork	3 ounces	303	171
Tofu, raw, firm, prepared with calcium sulfate	1/2 cup	299	181
Haddock	3 ounces	298	77
Beef	3 ounces	288	173
Pistachio nuts	1 ounce	286	162
Deer	3 ounces	285	134
Lamb	3 ounces	285	158
Salmon (various)	3 ounces	~280–535	~115–175
Game meats (various)	3 ounces	~285–345	~115–180
Other Sources			
Coconut water, unsweetened	1 cup	396	43

[a] All foods listed are assumed to be in nutrient-dense forms; lean or low-fat and prepared with minimal added sugars, saturated fat, or sodium.

[b] Some fortified foods and beverages are included. Other fortified options may exist on the market, but not all fortified foods are nutrient-dense. For example, some foods with added sugars may be fortified and would not be examples in the lists provided here.

[c] Some foods or beverages are not appropriate for all ages (eg, nuts, raw carrots), particularly young children for whom some foods could be a choking hazard.

[d] Portions listed are not recommended serving sizes.

[e] Seafood varieties include choices from the US Food and Drug Administration and US Environmental Protection Agency joint "Advice About Eating Fish," available at FDA.gov/fishadvice and EPA.gov/fishadvice from the "Best Choices" list. Varieties from the "Best Choices" list that contain even lower methylmercury include flatfish (eg, flounder), salmon, tilapia, shrimp, catfish, crab, trout, haddock, oysters, sardines, squid, pollock, anchovies, crawfish, mullet, scallops, whiting, clams, shad, and Atlantic mackerel.

Data Source: US Department of Agriculture, Agricultural Research Service. FoodData Central, 2019. fdc.nal.usda.gov.

Adapted from US Department of Agriculture, US Department of Health and Human Services. Food sources of potassium. Dietary Guidelines for Americans. Accessed March 20, 2023. https://www.dietaryguidelines.gov/food-sources-potassium.

Saturated and Polyunsaturated Fat and Cholesterol Content of Common Foods

Food	Quantity	Saturated Fat, g	Polyunsaturated Fat, g	Cholesterol, mg	Kilocalories
Almonds (roasted, salted, shelled)	1 ounce	1.2	3.7	0	170
Avocado	1 cup	3.0	2.7	0	240
Bacon (cured, cooked)	2 slices	2.3	0.8	17	89
Beef, lean, choice	3 ounces	2.9	0.4	76	175
Bread, white	1 slice	0.2	0.5	0	77
Butter	1 tablespoon	7.3	0.4	31	102
Cheese					
Cheddar	1 ounce	5.4	0.4	28	115
Cottage, creamed	½ cup	1.9	0.1	19	111
Cream or spread	2 tablespoons	5.9	0.4	29	102
Chicken (breast meat, without skin)	3½ ounces	1.0	0.8	84	164
Coconut (dried, sweetened)	¼ cup	7.3	0.1	0	116
Canola oil	1 tablespoon	1.0	3.9	0	124
Coconut oil	1 tablespoon	11.2	0.2	0	121
Corn oil	1 tablespoon	1.8	7.4	0	122
Egg					
Whole, hard-boiled	1 large	1.6	0.7	186	78
White	1 large	0	0	0	17
Yolk	1 large	1.6	0.7	184	55
Fish (fillet or flounder, sole)	3 ounces	0.5	0.4	48	73
Hamburger (85% lean)	3 ounces	5.0	0.4	75	212
Ice cream (light) vanilla	½ cup	2.2	0.2	21	137
Lamb (lean, leg)	3 ounces	2.4	0.4	76	162
Lard	1 tablespoon	5.0	1.4	12	115
Liver (beef)	3½ ounces	2.9	1.1	393	192
Margarine					
Regular (hydrogenated)	1 tablespoon	2.4	3.0	0	101
Tub	1 tablespoon	2.0	3.8	0	101
Smart Beat Smart Squeeze	1 tablespoon	0.04	0.17	0	7
Milk					
Whole	1 cup	4.6	0.5	24	149
2%	1 cup	3.1	0.2	20	122
Skim	1 cup	0.1	0	5	83
Almond beverage, sweetened	1 cup	0	0.5	0	91
Soy beverage, fortified	1 cup	0.5	2.1	0	104
Olive oil	1 tablespoon	1.9	1.4	0	119
Oysters (eastern, wild-farmed)	6 medium	0.4	0.4–0.5	34–21	43–50
Pam Cooking Spray	3-s spray	0.05	0.2	0	7
Peanut oil	1 tablespoon	2.3	4.3	0	119
Pork (lean, loin)	3½ ounces	3.4	0.7	78	202

Adapted from American Academy of Pediatrics Committee on Nutrition. *Pediatric Nutrition.* Kleinman RE, Greer FR, eds. 8th ed. American Academy of Pediatrics; 2020:1617–1622.

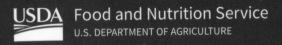
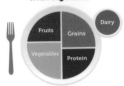

Rethink Fats

Healthy eating is important at every age. Eat a variety of fruits, vegetables, grains, protein foods, and dairy or fortified soy alternatives. When deciding what to eat or drink, choose options that are full of nutrients and limited in added sugars, saturated fat, and sodium. Start with these tips:

Check the label first

Read the Nutrition Facts label on packaged foods. Choose products that are lower in saturated fat since these types of fat are less healthy.

Eat foods with healthy fats

Eat nuts, seeds, and fatty fish like tuna, salmon, and sardines. These foods, as well as vegetable oils like olive and canola, are good sources of unsaturated fat—a healthier fat option.

Limit saturated fat

Build meals around protein foods that are naturally low in saturated fat such as beans, peas, and lentils, as well as soy foods, skinless chicken, seafood, and lean meats.

Skimp on "solid fats"

"Solid fats" such as butter, shortening, and fat from meats are high in saturated fats. Switch to olive or canola oil for cooking and trim the fat when possible.

Swap the spread

Switch from butter and cream cheese on your toast to a nut butter or a spread of avocado and a squeeze of lemon. These spread options contain healthier fats.

Customize your order

Order baked or steamed options instead of fried foods, especially deep-fried foods. A dash of hot sauce or a spoonful of salsa adds flavor without adding fat.

Go to **MyPlate**.gov for more information.
USDA is an equal opportunity provider, employer, and lender.

The benefits of healthy eating add up over time, bite by bite.

FNS-905-8
March 2022

TAB 18

Beverages and Milk

Comparison of Common Unflavored Milk Alternatives

	Whole Milk (1 cup [240 mL])	Rice Beverage (1 cup [240 mL])	Soy Beverage (1 cup [240 mL])	Coconut Milk (1 cup [240 mL])	Almond Beverage (1 cup [240 mL])	Oat Beverage (1 cup [240 mL])	Hemp Beverage (1 cup [240 mL])	Pea Beverage (1 cup [240 mL])
Energy (kcal)	149	115	105	76	37	130	70	80
Protein (g)	7.69	0.68	6.34	0.51	1.44	4	3	8
Total fat (g)	7.93	2.37	3.59	5.08	2.68	2.5	5	4.5
Saturated fat (g)	4.55	0	0.5	5.083	0	0	0.5	0.5
Cholesterol (mg)	24	0	0	0	0	0	0	0
Carbohydrate (g)	11.71	22.37	12	7.12	1.42	24	1	<1
Calcium (mg)	276	288	300	459	481	350	300	440
Iron (mg)	0.07	0.49	1.02	0.73	0.85	1.8	1.8	0
Vitamin D (IU)	128	96	108	96	96	100	100	110

Note: Homemade almond "milk" or other homemade "milk" alternatives do not contain the same number of vitamins, because they are not fortified.

From Porto A, Drake R. Cow's milk alternatives: parent FAQs. HealthyChildren.org. Updated June 2, 2022. Accessed March 20, 2023. https://www.healthychildren.org/English/healthy-living/nutrition/Pages/milk-allergy-foods-and-ingredients-to-avoid.aspx.

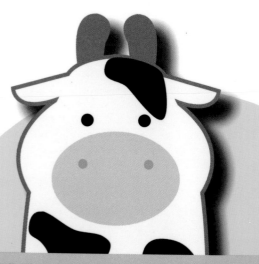

Suggested Daily Water and Milk Intake for Infants and Young Children

	6–12 months	12–24 months	2–5 years
Water	4–8 oz/day 0.5–1 cup/day	8–32 oz/day 1–4 cups/day	8–40 oz/day 1–5 cups/day
Cow's milk[a]	None	16–24 oz/day 2–3 cups/day	16–20 oz/day 2–2.5 cups/day

[a] Children ages 12–24 months are advised to drink whole milk and children 2 and older nonfat (skim) or low-fat (1%) milk.

From Muth MD. Recommended drinks for children age 5 and younger. HealthyChildren.org. Updated May 13, 2022. Accessed March 21, 2023. https://www.healthychildren.org/English/healthy-living/nutrition/Pages/Recommended-Drinks-for-Young-Children-Ages-0-5.aspx.

Nondairy Alternative Fortification Requirements

Nutrient	Per Cup (8 fl oz)
Calcium	276 mg
Protein	8 g
Vitamin A	500 IU
Vitamin D	100 IU
Magnesium	24 mg
Phosphorus	222 mg
Potassium	349 mg
Riboflavin	0.44 mg
Vitamin B$_{12}$	1.1 µg

From American Academy of Pediatrics Committee on Nutrition. *Pediatric Nutrition.* Kleinman RE, Greer FR, eds. 8th ed. American Academy of Pediatrics; 2020:248.

TAB 18

Beverages and Milk

Calories and Electrolytes in Beverages

Calories and Selected Electrolytes (per fl oz)				
Beverage	Energy, kcal	Sodium, mg	Potassium, mg	Phosphorous, mg
Regular Soft Drinks				
Cola or pepper cola	13	1–3	0–2	3
Decaffeinated cola	13	1	2	3
Lemon-lime (clear)	12	3	0	0
Orange	15	4	1	0
Grape	13	5	0	0
Root beer	13	4	0	0
Ginger ale	10	2	0	0
Tonic water	10	2	0	0
Diet Soft Drinks				
Diet cola or pepper cola	1	1–2	2	3
Decaffeinated diet cola or pepper cola	0	1	2	3
Diet lemon-lime	0	2	1	0
Diet root beer	0	5	3	1
Club soda, seltzer, and sparkling water	0	6	1	0
Juices				
Apricot nectar, canned	18	1	36	3
Apple juice, unsweetened	14	1	31	2
Cranberry juice cocktail, bottled	17	1	4	0
Cranberry juice (100% juice)	14	2	23	2
Cranberry juice, diet	1	2	2	0
Fruit punch	15	12	10	1
Grape juice, canned, unsweetened	19	2	33	4
Grapefruit juice, canned, unsweetened	12	0	47	3

Calories and Selected Electrolytes (per fl oz)				
Beverage	Energy, kcal	Sodium, mg	Potassium, mg	Phosphorous, mg
Juices (continued)				
Orange juice, with or without pulp	15	1	55	15
Pear nectar, canned	19	1	4	1
Peach nectar, canned	17	2	12	2
Pineapple juice, canned, unsweetened	17	1	41	3
Pomegranate juice	17	3	67	3
Strawberry and watermelon blend Juicy Juice	15	2	34	0
Tomato juice, canned, without salt added	5	3	70	5
Sports (Electrolyte) Drinks				
Gatorade	7	12	5	3
Powerade	10	13	5	0
G2	2	13	4	2
Powerade Zero	0	13	3	0
Vitamin Water Zero	0	0	44	0
Pedialyte	3	32	24	3
Caffeinated Drinks				
Coffee	0	1	15	1
Tea	0	1	11	0
Iced coffee (mocha, milk-based)	20	10	45	20
Iced tea, bottled, unsweetened	0	1	0	0
Iced tea, sweetened	11	6	6	8
Sweetened tea beverage (AriZona, Arnold Palmer)	12	1	3	0
Energy drink	14	3	1	0

Adapted from American Academy of Pediatrics Committee on Nutrition. *Pediatric Nutrition*. Kleinman RE, Greer FR, eds. 8th ed. American Academy of Pediatrics; 2020:1563–1566. From Nutrient Data Laboratory, Agricultural Research Service, US Department of Agriculture. USDA National Nutrient Database for Standard Reference. Release 28. Updated May 24, 2022. Accessed March 21, 2023. https://data.nal.usda.gov/dataset/composition-foods-raw-processed-prepared-usda-national-nutrient-database-standard-reference-release-28-0.

TAB 19

Vitamin Deficiency

Vitamin Deficiency States, Recommended Intake, Deficiency Symptoms, Deficiency Risk Factors, Diagnostic Tests, and Therapeutic Dosages

Nutrient	Recommended Intake	Deficiency Name	Deficiency Symptoms	Deficiency Risk Factors	Diagnostic Tests	Food Sources	Recommended Therapeutic Dosage
Vitamin A	RDA 1–18 y: 1–3 y 1,000 IU/day 4–8 y 1,430 IU/day 9–13 y 2,000 IU/day 14–18 y 2,310–3,000 IU/day		Night blindness, infection (measles), keratomalacia	Fat malabsorption	Serum retinol Serum retinol-binding protein	Liver, eggs, dairy, vegetables	100,000–200,000 IU, orally
Vitamin D	>1 y 600 IU/day	Rickets	Rickets, hypocalcemia, tetany, osteomalacia, hypophosphatemia	Fat malabsorption, lack of sunshine	Radiography, serum 25-OH-D	Fatty fish egg yolk	2,000–5,000 IU/day
Vitamin E	RDA all ages: 1–3 y 6 mg/day 4–8 y 7 mg/day 9–13 y 11 mg/day 14–18 y 15 mg/day		Neuropathy, ataxia	Fat malabsorption	Serum α-tocopherol	Grain and vegetable oils	25 IU/kg/day for fat malabsorption
Vitamin K	AI all ages: 1–3 y 30 µg/day 4–8 y 55 µg/day 9–18 y 60–75 µg/day		Bleeding	Fat malabsorption, breastfeeding	PT, PIVKA, clotting factors	Green vegetables, soy oil, seeds, fruits	1 mg, intramuscularly, in newborn infants
Thiamine (B$_1$)	RDA 1–18 y: 1–3 y 0.5 mg/day 4–8 y 0.6 mg/day 9–13 y 0.9 mg/day 14–18 y 1–1.2 mg/day	Beriberi or Wernicke encephalopathy	Beriberi: symmetrical, peripheral neuropathy, edema; Wernicke: ophthalmoplegia, nystagmus, ataxia	HIV, alcohol abuse, dialysis, gastrointestinal tract disease, TPN, anorexia, furosemide, food faddism; inflammation in pediatric intensive care unit	Whole blood/RBC transketolase activation test, baseline and after TPP; or TPP level, urinary total thiamine	Unrefined grain, liver, pork, vegetables, dairy, peanuts, legumes, fruits, eggs	Severe infantile: 50–100 mg parenteral × 1 Children: 10–25 mg/day parenteral × 2 wk, followed by 5–10 mg/day, orally, × 1 mo Mild: 10 mg/day, orally, until resolution
Riboflavin (B$_2$)	RDA 1–18 y: 1–3 y 0.5 mg/day 4–8 y 0.6 mg/day 9–13 y 0.9 mg/day 14–18 y 1–1.3 mg/day		Pharyngitis, cheilosis, angular stomatitis, glossitis, seborrheic dermatitis	Weaning from breast-feeding, breastfed from deficient mother, alcoholism, phototherapy, cystic fibrosis, malnutrition, thyroid insufficiency, adrenal insufficiency	RBC or 24-h urine riboflavin level or RBC glutathione reductase (but of limited value in glutathione reductase deficiency, G6PD deficiency, or β-thalassemia)	Milk, cheese, eggs, liver, lean meats, green vegetables	Infants: 0.5 mg, orally, twice/wk Children: 1 mg, orally, dose 3×/day until resolution
Niacin (B$_3$)	RDA 1–18 y: 1–3 y 6 mg/day 4–8 y 8 mg/day 9–13 y 12 mg/day 14–18 y 14–16 mg/day	Pellagra	Diarrhea, dermatitis, dementia, glossitis, angular stomatitis, sun-exposed	Crohn disease; anorexia nervosa; Hartnup disease; Carcinoid syndrome; immigrant from area with nonfortified grains; medications isoniazid, anticonvulsants, antidepressants, 5-fluorouracil, 6-mercaptopurine, chloramphenicol, sulfas	24-h niacin and N-methylnicotinamide; or RBC NAD/NADP niacin number	Beef, liver, fish, pork, wheat flour, eggs	50–100 mg/dose, orally, 3×/day for several wks

TAB 19

Vitamin Deficiency

Vitamin Deficiency States, Recommended Intake, Deficiency Symptoms, Deficiency Risk Factors, Diagnostic Tests, and Therapeutic Dosages (*continued*)

Nutrient	Recommended Intake	Deficiency Name	Deficiency Symptoms	Deficiency Risk Factors	Diagnostic Tests	Food Sources	Recommended Therapeutic Dosage
Pantothenic acid (B₅)	AI all ages: 1–3 y 2 mg/day 4–8 y 3 mg/day 9–13 y 4 mg/day 14–18 y 5 mg/day		Not characterized		24-h pantothenic acid	Chicken, beef, potatoes, oats, tomatoes, liver, kidney, yeast, egg yolk, broccoli	
Pyridoxine (B₆)	RDA 1–18 y: 1–3 y 0.5 mg/day 4–8 y 0.6 mg/day 9–13 y 1 mg/day 14–18 y 1.2–1.3 mg/day		Glossitis, cheilosis, angular stomatitis, depression, confusion	Chronic renal failure, leukemia; pyridoxine-dependent seizure; alcoholism; medications isoniazid, hydralazine, penicillamine, theophylline	Plasma pyridoxal 5'-phosphate; 24-h urine 4-pyridoxic acid	Meat, liver, kidneys	Without neuropathy: 5–25 mg orally/day × 3 wk With neuropathy: 10–50 mg/day, orally, × 3 wk; then followed by 1.5–2.5 mg/day, orally Seizures: 50–100 mg, intravenously or intramuscularly
Biotin (B₇)	AI all ages: 1–3 y 8 µg/day 4–8 y 12 µg/day 9–13 y 20 µg/day 14–18 y 25 µg/day		Hypotonia, exfoliative dermatitis	Infants with TPN without biotin, eating large amounts of undercooked eggs, holo-carboxylase synthase deficiency, biotinidase deficiency, biotin transport defect, anticonvulsants	Urinary biotin or urinary 3-hydroxyisovaleric acid; lymphocyte propionyl-CoA carboxylase concentration, or leukocyte LSC19A3 transporter	Chard, tomatoes, romaine lettuce, carrots	Acquired deficiency: 150 µg/day
Folate (B₉)	RDA 1–18 y: 1–3 y 150 µg/day 4–8 y 200 µg/day 9–13 y 300 µg/day 14–18 y 400 µg/day		Megaloblastic anemia, neural tube defect, cleft lip/palate	Poor intakes relatively common at 12 mo; consuming carbonated beverages; Crohn disease; fruit and carb; diarrhea; HIV, familial; medications methotrexate, trimethoprim, oral contraceptives, pyrimethamine, phenobarbital, phenytoin	Plasma or serum folate (acute); RBC folate (chronic deficiency); 5-methyltetrahydrofolate; or urinary total folate	Cauliflower, green vegetables, yeast, liver, kidney	Children 1–13: 1 mg/day, followed by 0.1–0.5 mg/day Children >13: 1 mg/day
Cobalamin (B₁₂)	RDA 1–18 y: 1–3 y 0.9 µg/day 4–8 y 1.2 µg/day 9–13 y 1.8 µg/day 14–18 y 2.4 µg/day		Megaloblastic anemia, ataxia, muscle weakness, spasticity, incontinence, hypotension, vision problems, dementia, psychosis, mood disturbance, neural tube defect	Breastfed children of strict vegans; post bariatric surgery or stomach or ileal resection; pernicious anemia; bacterial overgrowth of gut; phenylketonuria; Whipple disease; Zollinger-Ellison syndrome; celiac disease; medications H₂ blockers	Serum cobalamin concentration, plasma homocysteine or serum methyl-malonic acid in PKU patient	Fish, eggs, cheese	Children: 30–50 µg/day, intramuscularly, × 2 wk, followed by 100 µg, intramuscularly, every mo, or 1 mg orally/day
Vitamin C	RDA 1–18 y: 1–3 y 15 mg/day 4–8 y 25 mg/day 9–13 y 45 mg/day 14–18 y 65–75 mg/day	Scurvy	Osmotic diarrhea, bleeding gums, arthropathy, perifollicular hemorrhage	Overcooked foods, with minimal fruits and vegetables, anorexia nervosa, autism, ulcerative colitis, Whipple disease, dialysis, alcoholics, tobacco, TPN without vitamin C	White blood cell ascorbate concentration, urinary ascorbate, capillary fragility, widening of zone of provisional calcification bone ends on radiographs	Citrus fruits	Children: 25–100 mg, orally, intramuscularly, or intravenously, 3×/day × 1 wk, followed by 100 mg orally/day

AI indicates adequate intake; CoA, coenzyme A; G6PD, glucose-6-phosphate dehydrogenase; PIVKA, proteins induced by vitamin K absence; PKU, phenylketonuria; PT, prothrombin time; RBC, red blood cell; RDA, recommended dietary allowance; TPN, total parenteral nutrition; and TPP, thiamine pyrophosphate.

Adapted from American Academy of Pediatrics Committee on Nutrition. *Pediatric Nutrition*. Kleinman RE, Greer FR, eds. 8th ed. American Academy of Pediatrics; 2020:626–631.

TAB 20

Picky Eating/Feeding Difficulties

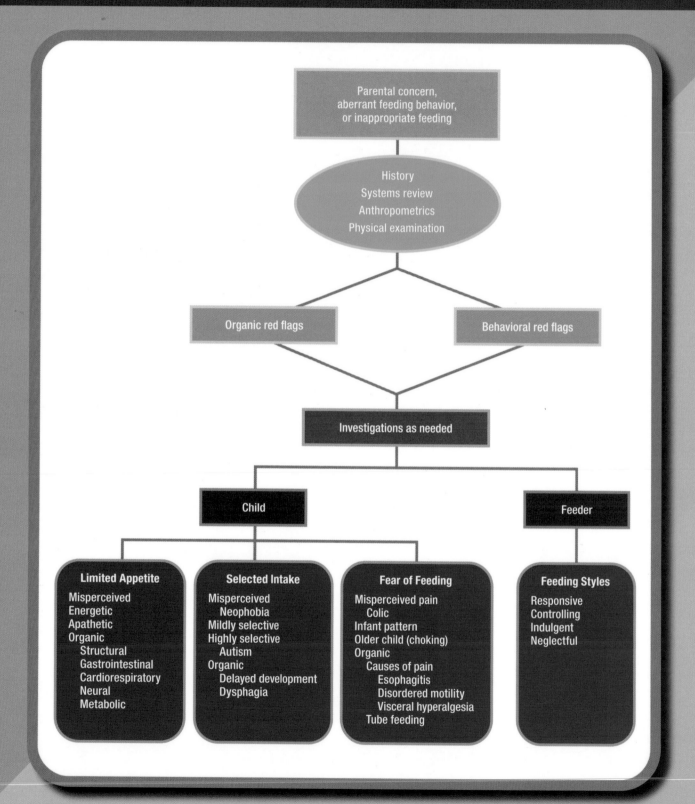

An approach to identifying and managing feeding difficulties.

From Kerzner B, Milano K, MacLean WC Jr, Berall G, Stuart S, Chatoor I. A practical approach to classifying and managing feeding difficulties. *Pediatrics.* 2015;135(2):346.

Presenting Features of Feeding Difficulties

Suggestive symptoms/signs	Prolonged mealtimes
	Food refusal lasting < 1 mo
	Disruptive and stressful mealtimes
	Lack of appropriate independent feeding
	Nocturnal eating in toddler
	Distraction to increase intake
	Prolonged breast- or bottle-feeding
	Failure to advance textures
Organic red flags[a]	Dysphagia
	Aspiration
	Apparent pain with feeding
	Vomiting and diarrhea
	Developmental delay
	Chronic cardio-respiratory symptoms
	Growth failure (failure to thrive)
Behavioral red flags[a]	Food fixation (selective, extreme dietary limitations)
	Noxious (forceful and/or persecutory) feeding
	Abrupt cessation of feeding after a trigger event
	Anticipatory gagging
	Failure to thrive

[a] Red flags are signs/symptoms that require prompt attention and, in many instances, referral for in-depth investigation or specialized treatment.

Adapted from Kerzner B, Milano K, MacLean WC Jr, Berall G, Stuart S, Chatoor I. A practical approach to classifying and managing feeding difficulties. *Pediatrics.* 2015;135(2):346.

Criteria for an "ideal" classification of feeding difficulties

Feeding difficulties can be classified based on parents' expressed concerns about their child's feeding/eating behavior, which fall into 3 principal categories: those not eating enough (limited appetite); those eating an inadequate variety of foods (selective intake); and those afraid to eat (fear of feeding). Each category has subcategories to acknowledge that such concerns may be a misperception on the part of the parents or primarily behavioral or organic, both with a spectrum ranging from mild to severe.

➡ The criteria for an "ideal" classification of feeding difficulties systematically categorize the following:
  – Behavioral issues
  – Organic conditions
  – Caregiver feeding styles

➡ The criteria are used to separate misperceived, mild, and severe conditions.

➡ Conditions can therefore be
  – Readily recognized
  – Identified by familiar and accurate terminology
  – Logically related to each other
  – Manageable in number

➡ Specific treatment options are available for each condition.

Adapted from Kerzner B, Milano K, MacLean WC Jr, Berall G, Stuart S, Chatoor I. A practical approach to classifying and managing feeding difficulties. *Pediatrics.* 2015;135(2):347.

Feeding guidelines for all children

Reviewing the following basic feeding guidelines with parents can be useful when managing a child with a limited appetite:

➡ Avoid distractions during mealtimes (television, cell phones, etc)

➡ Maintain a pleasant neutral attitude throughout meal

➡ Feed to encourage appetite
  – Limit meal duration (20–30 min)
  – 4–6 meals/snacks a day with only water in between

➡ Serve age-appropriate foods

➡ Systematically introduce new foods (up to 8–15 times)

➡ Encourage self-feeding

➡ Tolerate age-appropriate mess

Adapted from Kerzner B, Milano K, MacLean WC Jr, Berall G, Stuart S, Chatoor I. A practical approach to classifying and managing feeding difficulties. *Pediatrics.* 2015;135(2):347.

TAB 21

Malnutrition

Key Domains for Defining Pediatric Nutrition

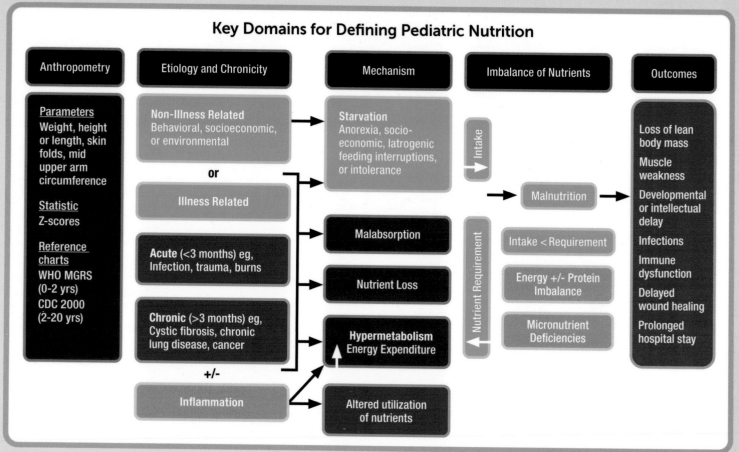

CDC indicates Centers for Disease Control and Prevention; MGRS, Multicentre Growth Reference Study; and WHO, World Health Organization. +/- indicates with or without.

Reprinted with permission from Mehta NM, Corkins MR, Lyman B, et al; American Society for Parenteral and Enteral Nutrition Board of Directors. Defining pediatric malnutrition: a paradigm shift toward etiology-related definitions. *JPEN J Parenter Enteral Nutr.* 2013;37(4):460–481.

Patients at high risk for malnutrition

- ➤ Patients with malnutrition or evidence of cachexia present at diagnosis
- ➤ Patients expected to receive highly emetogenic regimens
- ➤ Patients treated with regimens associated with severe gastrointestinal complications such as constipation, diarrhea, loss of appetite, mucositis, enterocolitis
- ➤ Patients with relapsed disease
- ➤ Patients who are < 2 months old
- ➤ Patients who are expected to receive radiation to the oropharynx/esophagus or abdomen
- ➤ Patients on chemotherapy treatment protocols with high occurrence of gastrointestinal or appetite-depressing effects such as those for Burkitt lymphoma, osteogenic sarcoma, and central nervous system tumors
- ➤ Patients with postsurgical complications such as prolonged ileus or short gut syndrome
- ➤ Patients receiving a hematopoietic stem cell transplant
- ➤ Patients with inadequate availability of nutrients because of low socioeconomic status

From American Academy of Pediatrics Committee on Nutrition. *Pediatric Nutrition.* Kleinman RE, Greer FR, eds. 8th ed. American Academy of Pediatrics; 2020:1154.

TAB 21

Malnutrition

Diagnostic Criteria for Undernutrition

	Severe Acute Malnutrition	Moderate Acute Malnutrition	Stunting	Underweight
Weight-for-age	NA	NA	NA	Less than −2 SD
Height-for-age (or length-for-age)	NA	NA	Less than −2 SD	NA
Weight-for-height (or weight-for-length)	Less than −3 SD	Between −2 SD and −3 SD	NA	NA
Mid-upper arm circumference	< 11.5 cm	Between 11.5 and 12.5 cm	NA	NA
Edema	+/−	No	No	NA

NA indicates not applicable. +/- indicates with or without.

From American Academy of Pediatrics Committee on Nutrition. *Pediatric Nutrition.* Kleinman RE, Greer FR, eds. 8th ed. American Academy of Pediatrics; 2020:275.

Classification of Malnutrition in Adolescents and Young Adults With Eating Disorders (*See Tab 22*)

	Mild	Moderate	Severe
BMI, median, %	80–90	70–79	<70
BMI *z* score	−1.0 to −1.9	−2.0 to −2.9	≥−3.0
Weight loss	>10% Body mass loss	>15% Body mass loss	>20% Body mass loss in 1 year or >10% body mass loss in 6 months

BMI indicates body mass index.

This is a proposed classification of degree of malnutrition in adolescents and young adults with eating disorders as reported in the Society for Adolescent Health and Medicine position paper on medical management of restrictive eating disorders in adolescents and young adults.

Adapted from Seetharaman S, Fields EL. Avoidant/restrictive food intake disorder. *Ped Rev.* 2020;41(12):617.

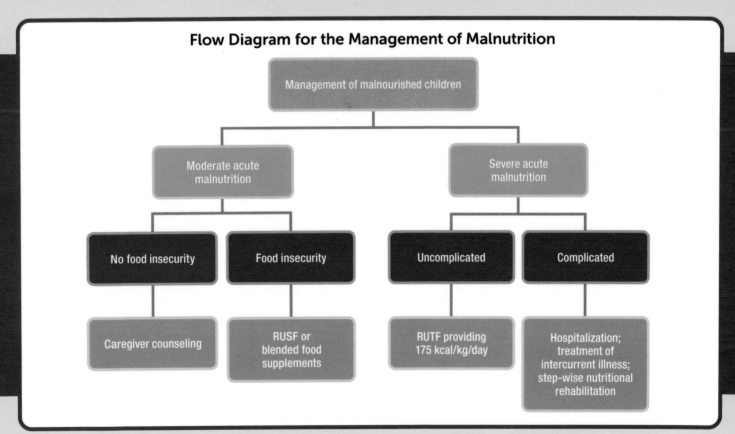

Flow Diagram for the Management of Malnutrition

RUSF indicates ready-to-use supplementary food; RUTF, ready-to-use therapeutic food. For more information about food insecurity, see Tab 23.

From American Academy of Pediatrics Committee on Nutrition. *Pediatric Nutrition.* Kleinman RE, Greer FR, eds. 8th ed. American Academy of Pediatrics; 2020:278.

TAB 22

Eating Disorders

Diagnostic Features of Eating Disorders Commonly Seen in Children and Adolescents

Anorexia Nervosa (AN)

Restricted caloric intake relative to energy requirements, leading to significantly low body weight for age, sex, projected growth, and physical health

Intense fear of gaining weight or behaviors that consistently interfere with weight gain, despite being at a significantly low weight

Altered perception of one's body weight or shape, excessive influence of body weight or shape on self-value, or persistent lack of acknowledgment of the seriousness of one's low body weight

Subtypes: restricting type (weight loss is achieved primarily through dieting, fasting, and/or excessive exercise. In the previous 3 months, there have been no repeated episodes of binge eating or purging); binge-eating/purging type (in the previous 3 months, there have been repeated episodes of binge eating or purging; ie, self-induced vomiting or misuse of laxatives, diuretics, or enemas)

Atypical AN

Restricted caloric intake relative to energy requirements, with weight normal, obese, or overweight despite this limited intake

Intense fear of gaining weight or behaviors that consistently interfere with weight gain, despite being at a significantly low weight

All of the criteria for AN are met, yet the individual's weight is within or above the normal range despite significant weight loss

Subtypes: none in the *DSM-5*

Bulimia Nervosa (BN)

Repeated episodes of binge eating. Binge eating is characterized by both of the following: within a distinct period of time (eg, 2 hours), eating an amount of food that is larger than what most individuals would eat during a similar period of time under similar circumstances and a sense that one cannot limit or control their overeating during the episode

Repeated use of inappropriate compensatory behaviors for the prevention of weight gain, such as self-induced vomiting; misuse of laxatives, diuretics, or other medications; fasting; or excessive exercise

On average, the binge eating and compensatory behaviors both occur at least once a week for 3 months

Self-value is overly influenced by body shape and weight

The binge eating and compensatory behaviors do not occur exclusively during episodes of AN

Subthreshold BN

BN (of low frequency and/or limited duration): All of the criteria for BN are met, but, on average, the binge eating and compensatory behaviors occur less than once a week and/or for <3 months

Binge-Eating Disorder (BED)

Recurrent episodes of binge eating. An episode of binge eating is characterized by both of the following: within a distinct period of time (eg, 2 hours), eating an amount of food that is clearly larger than what most individuals would eat during a similar period of time under similar circumstances and sense that one cannot limit or control their overeating during the episode

The binge-eating episodes include 3 or more of the following: eating much more quickly than normal, eating until uncomfortably full, eating large amounts of food when not feeling hungry, eating alone because of embarrassment at how much one is eating, and feeling guilty, disgusted, or depressed afterward

Marked anguish is experienced regarding binge eating

On average, the binge eating occurs at least once a week for 3 months

The binge eating is not associated with the use of inappropriate compensatory behavior as in BN and does not occur only in the context of BN or AN

BED of Low Frequency

BED (of low frequency and/or limited duration): All of the criteria for BED are met, but, on average, the binge eating occurs less than once a week and/or for <3 months

Avoidant/Restrictive Food Intake Disorder (ARFID)

A disrupted eating pattern (eg, seeming lack of interest in eating or food; avoidance based on the sensory qualities of food; concern about unpleasant consequences of eating) as evidenced by persistent failure to meet appropriate nutritional and/or energy needs associated with 1 (or more) of the following: significant weight loss or, in children, failure to achieve expected growth and/or weight gain, marked nutritional deficiency, reliance on enteral feeding or oral nutritional supplements, significant interference with psychosocial functioning

The disturbance cannot be better explained by lack of available food or by an associated culturally sanctioned practice

The eating disturbance cannot be attributed to a coexisting medical condition nor better explained by another mental disorder. If the eating disturbance occurs in the context of another condition or disorder, the severity of the eating disturbance exceeds that routinely associated with the condition or disorder

Other Specified Feeding or Eating Disorders, Examples

Purging disorder: recurrent purging behavior (eg, self-induced vomiting; misuse of laxatives, diuretics, or other medications) in the absence of binge eating with the intent to influence weight or body shape

DSM-5 indicates *Diagnostic and Statistical Manual of Mental Disorders, Fifth Edition*. Adapted from Hornberger LL, Lane MA; American Academy of Pediatrics Committee on Adolescence. Identification and management of eating disorders in children and adolescents. *Pediatrics*. 2021;147(1):e2.

TAB 22

Eating Disorders

Differential Diagnosis of Eating Disorders

Diagnosis	Clinical Features
Vomiting	
Chronic cholecystitis	Constant right upper quadrant pain
CNS lesion	Headache, seizure, visual disturbances
Pancreatitis	Persistent, severe epigastric abdominal pain
Pregnancy	Amenorrhea, fatigue, (+) pregnancy test result
Superior mesenteric artery syndrome	Postprandial epigastric pain with early satiety, bilious emesis
Weight Loss	
Adrenal insufficiency	Postural dizziness, hypotension, hyperkalemia, hypercalcemia, hyponatremia
Celiac disease	Chronic diarrhea with foul-smelling and/or floating stools, constipation with abdominal distention
Depression	Anhedonia, ⬇appetite, sleep disturbance, feelings of worthlessness or guilt, impaired concentration
Diabetes mellitus	Polyuria, polydipsia, hyperglycemia
HIV	Fever, lymphadenopathy, sore throat, mucocutaneous ulcer, rash, myalgia, night sweats, diarrhea
Hyperthyroidism	Anxiety, emotional lability, weakness, tremor, palpitations, heat intolerance, ⬆perspiration
Inflammatory bowel disease	Bloody diarrhea, colicky abdominal pain, urgency, tenesmus, incontinence, hypotension
Substance use	Needle marks, skin infections, unexplained burns, atrophy of nasal mucosa

CNS indicates central nervous system. (+) indicates a positive finding; ⬇, decreased; and ⬆, increased.
From American Academy of Pediatrics Section on Hospital Medicine. *Caring for the Hospitalized Child: A Handbook of Inpatient Pediatrics.* Gershel JC, Rausch DA, eds. 3rd ed. American Academy of Pediatrics; 2023:13.

Eating disorders: when hospitalization is needed

One or more of the following justify hospitalization:

1. ≤75% median body mass index for age and sex
2. Dehydration
3. Electrolyte disturbance (hypokalemia, hyponatremia, hypophosphatemia)
4. Electrocardiographic abnormalities (eg, prolonged QTc or severe bradycardia)
5. Physiological instability
   a. Severe bradycardia (heart rate <50 beats/minute daytime; <45 beats/minute at night)
   b. Hypotension (<90/45 mm Hg)
   c. Hypothermia (body temperature <96°F [35.6°C])
   d. Orthostatic increase in pulse (>20 beats per minute) or decrease in blood pressure (>20 mm Hg systolic or >10 mm Hg diastolic)
6. Arrested growth and development
7. Failure of outpatient treatment
8. Acute food refusal
9. Uncontrollable bingeing and purging
10. Acute medical complications of malnutrition (eg, syncope, seizures, cardiac failure, pancreatitis, etc)
11. Comorbid psychiatric or medical condition that prohibits or limits appropriate outpatient treatment (eg, severe depression, obsessive compulsive disorder, type 1 diabetes mellitus)

From American Academy of Pediatrics Committee on Nutrition. *Pediatric Nutrition.* Kleinman RE, Greer FR, eds. 8th ed. American Academy of Pediatrics; 2020:1091.

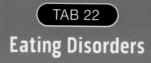

Screening for Disordered Eating: Example Questions to Ask Adolescents

History/Information	Example Questions
Weight history	What was your highest weight? How tall were you? How old were you?
	What was your lowest weight? How tall were you? How old were you?
Body image	What do you think your weight should be? What feels too high? What feels too low?
	Are there body areas that cause you stress? Which areas?
	Do you do any body checking (ie, weighing, body pinching or checking, mirror checking)?
	How much of your day is spent thinking about food or your body?
Diet history	24-hour diet history.
	Do you count calories, fat, carbohydrates? How much do you allow? What foods do you avoid?
	Do you ever feel guilty about eating? How do you deal with that guilt (ie, exercising, purging, eating less)?
	Do you feel out of control when eating?
Exercise history	Do you exercise? What activities? How often? How intense is your workout?
	How stressed do you feel when you are unable to exercise?
Binge eating and purging	Do you ever binge? On what foods? How much? How often? Any triggers?
	Do you vomit? How often? How soon after eating?
	Do you use laxatives, diuretics, diet pills, caffeine? What types? How many? How often?
Family history	Does anyone in your family have a history of dieting or an eating disorder? Anyone on special diets (eg, vegetarian, gluten-free)? Anyone with obesity?
	Does anyone in your family have a history of depression, anxiety, bipolar disorder, obsessive-compulsive disorder, substance abuse, or other psychiatric illness?
	Does anyone in your family take psychiatric medication?
Review of systems	Dizziness, syncope, weakness or fatigue?
	Pallor, easy bruising or bleeding, cold intolerance?
	Hair loss, lanugo (extra hair growth on trunk, face, or extremities; the body's attempt to provide an extra layer of warmth in the face of starvation), dry skin?
	Constipation, diarrhea, early fullness, bloating, abdominal pain, heartburn?
	Palpitations, chest pain?
	Muscle cramps, joint pains?
	Excessive thirst and voiding?
	For girls: Age at menarche? Frequency of menses? LMP? Weight at time of LMP?

TAB 22

Eating Disorders

Screening for Disordered Eating: Example Questions to Ask Adolescents (*continued*)

History/Information	Example Questions
Psychosocial History (HEADSS)	
Home	Who lives in the home?
	How well do the family members get along with each other?
	Is the family experiencing any stressors?
Education	Where do you attend school? What grade? Regular classroom?
	Is school challenging for you? What grades do you receive? Has there been a change in your grades?
Activities	What activities are you involved in outside of the classroom?
	Do you have friends you can trust? Have you experienced any bullying?
	What social media sites/websites do you most often visit when you go online? How much time is spent online each day?
Drug use	Have you ever used tobacco, e-cigarettes, alcohol, or drugs? Which ones? How much? How often? With alcohol, any blackouts or passouts?
	Have you ever used anabolic steroids or stimulants? Caffeine consumption? Other substances?
Depression/suicide	How is your mood? Increased irritability? Feelings of depression or hopelessness? Any anxiety or obsessive-compulsive thoughts or behaviors?
	Any history of cutting or self-injury?
	Have you ever wished you were dead? How often do you have these thoughts? When was the last time? Any thoughts of suicide? What methods have you imagined? Any attempts?
	History of physical, sexual, or emotional abuse?
	Any previous mental health care?
Sexual history	Do you feel that the gender you feel inside matches your body on the outside?
	Are you romantically or sexually attracted to guys, girls, or both? Not sure?
	Have you had any sexual contact with another person? If yes, was it with guys, girls, or both? Use of condoms? Use of contraceptives? History of pregnancy or sexually transmitted infection?
	Has anyone done anything to you sexually that made you uncomfortable?

LMP indicates last menstrual period.

Adapted from Hornberger LL, Lane MA; American Academy of Pediatrics Committee on Adolescence. Identification and management of eating disorders in children and adolescents. *Pediatrics*. 2021;147(1):e2020040279. Originally adapted from Rome ES, Strandjord SE. Eating disorders. *Pediatr Rev.* 2016;37(8):323–336.

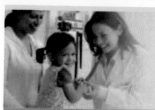

Hunger Vital Sign™

A validated tool to screen for food insecurity

Within the past 12 months, we worried whether our food would run out before we got money to buy more.

☐ Often true
☐ Sometimes true
☐ Never true

Within the past 12 months, the food we bought just didn't last and we didn't have money to get more.

☐ Often true
☐ Sometimes true
☐ Never true

A patient or family **screens positive** for food insecurity if the response is "often true" or "sometimes true" to either or both of these statements.

FRAC
Food Research & Action Center

Learn more about screening for and addressing food insecurity in health care settings at FRAC.org

---

How Pediatric Practices Are Connecting Patients to Food and Nutrition Programs: The Pros and Cons of Various Models

Program	Pros	Cons
Supplemental Nutrition Assistance Program (SNAP) SNAP is the foundation of the food security safety net and helps low-income individuals and families buy food at supermarkets, farmers' markets, and other food retail outlets. Health providers can help patients apply for SNAP, often in conjunction with an application for Medicaid, or connect patients to a community partner.	Benefits are 100 percent federally funded and are available for all who qualify. SNAP is effective in reducing food insecurity and improving health outcomes. SNAP is available in every state and the District of Columbia. Some communities have programs that double SNAP benefits at participating farmers' markets and food retailers. Learn more about Double Up and SNAP Doubling.	Not every patient will be eligible for SNAP (eg, may be over-income, may not have requisite immigrant status). Benefits for these programs are not issued in a single day. Many families already are benefitting from SNAP, but may run out of benefits before the end of the month.
Child Nutrition Programs The main child nutrition programs are the Special Supplemental Nutrition Program for Women, Infants, and Children (WIC); child care meals; school meals; afterschool snacks and meals; and summer food. Health providers can either help families access these programs directly or refer families to community partners.	All programs—with the exception of WIC—are entitlement programs, so they can serve all eligible children without the need for additional federal appropriations. Programs not only reduce food insecurity, but also improve academic achievement, early childhood development, and encourage healthier eating. The new public charge rule does not apply to these programs.	Patients may not meet age requirements. There may be limited availability of summer and/or afterschool meals sites in some communities.

(continues)

Program	Pros	Cons
Food Shelf A health provider, often in partnership with a local food bank or as the result of an internal food drive, collects nonperishable food staples that are stored on site. Criteria varies for which patients get free food items and how often. **Grocery Bags** Through a partnership with a local food bank, health providers distribute bags of groceries to patients periodically, typically once a month. The medical team and/or the food bank partner determines criteria for which patients get free food items. **Gift Cards to Local Supermarket** Practitioners distribute gift cards to a local supermarket to families in need of immediate food assistance. The practice determines the criteria for which patients receive the cards.	Responds to immediate need. Supplements food available from the federal nutrition programs. Supports nutritional needs of households experiencing food insecurity that may not be eligible for SNAP (eg, over-income, cannot satisfy citizenship or permanent legal residency requirements) or WIC (eg, over-income, children more than 4 years old).	Requires funding. Reach may be limited. This model is not sustainable unless ongoing funding is secured. Space constraints. Staff time needed. Food may not be tailored to the nutritional needs or cultural preferences of patients. This doesn't build on programs (eg, SNAP and WIC) that integrate families with food insecurity into normal commercial channels.
Summer Meal Site Instead of referring children to summer meal sites that may or may not be conveniently located, some health providers are hosting their own summer meal sites. This allows patients 18 years old and younger access to up to 2 free meals in a safe and convenient setting. Meals must meet nutrition standards, be served in a group setting, and cannot be taken home. Sites get reimbursed for meals served as well as some of the administrative costs of the program.	There is a sustainable amount of federal funding available to cover meal costs and some administrative costs. This program supports children's nutritional needs. Providers can partner with in-house food services or with a community partner to implement the model. Providers can serve children in the surrounding community.	There is a need for dedicated staff (or volunteers) to run the meal program. There is a need for space to serve meals in a group setting. Free meals are not provided for parents. Not all medical practices will be located in low-income areas that are eligible to participate in the program.
Afterschool Meal Site Through available federal funding, health care providers are offering out-of-school time meals after school, on weekends, or during school holidays to children 18 years old and younger. Meals must meet nutrition standards, be served in a group setting, and cannot be taken home. Afterschool meal program sites are required to offer enrichment activities. For example, a site can offer a nutrition education class that highlights how the food served supports the nutrition of children.	There is a sustainable amount of federal funding available to cover meal costs and some administrative costs. This program supports children's nutritional needs. Providers can partner with in-house food services or a community partner to implement the model. Providers can serve children in the surrounding community. Children benefit from enrichment activities. The program can reach children on weekends, during school holidays, and after school.	There is a need for dedicated staff (or volunteers) to run the meal program and enrichment activities. There is a need for space to serve meals in a group setting. Free meals are not provided for parents. Not all medical practices will be located in low-income areas that are eligible to participate in the program.
Food Pharmacy Selected patients who screen positive for food insecurity are referred to a medical center's food pharmacy where they meet with a staffer—often a dietitian—who identifies what foods are indicated for treatment of their medical condition. The patient then selects indicated foods from the food pharmacy and receives referrals to return once a month for 6 months. The dietitian also can screen patients for SNAP and other federal nutrition resources. ProMedica in Ohio developed an innovative food pharmacy model and is working to expand it to other hospital settings.	This is integrated into the hospital services and some staffing costs may be covered. Existing personnel can help staff the clinic. There is a dietitian on hand to help connect patients to appropriate food selections based on existing medical conditions. This program connects patients to SNAP, WIC, and other nutrition resources. Nutrition services are included in the patient's medical records.	This program requires additional funding. This program requires partnership with a food bank or funding to secure food for the pharmacy. This program requires dedicated space. This program cannot serve every patient who screens positive for food insecurity.

How Pediatric Practices Are Connecting Patients to Food and Nutrition Programs: The Pros and Cons of Various Models (*continued*)

Program	Pros	Cons
Veggie Rx and Veggie Incentive Programs Typically, the Veggie Rx and Veggie Incentive programs provide targeted patients (eg, who screen positive for food insecurity, diabetes, or obesity) with a "prescription" that can be used like cash and redeemed for fresh produce. Some programs only allow participants to redeem their prescriptions at participating farmers' markets or provide fruit and veggie boxes on site, while others partner with both farmers' markets and grocery stores. The structure of the program and the value of the "prescription" patients receive varies depending on the model. Wholesome Wave's Fruit and Vegetable Prescription Program (FVRx) provides $1 per day per household member.	The program can provide targeted support to patients diagnosed with diet-related chronic diseases to access fruits and vegetables.	Dedicated funding is required for this program. Can only reach a small number of patients. Need proximity to participating farmers' markets, grocery stores, or both.
Farmers' Markets Across the country, more health practices and hospitals are bringing farmers' markets and Mobile Markets on site so patients and staff can access healthy, local food. This model can better support families facing food insecurity if the market is able to accept SNAP benefits, WIC cash value vouchers, and participates in the federal WIC Farmers' Market Nutrition Program (FMNP).	This model provides access to local produce. Many markets can accept federal nutrition program benefits. This model may offer nutrition education at the market.	Dedicated staff and funding are needed to help implement this model; this is less so if a local farmers' market or mobile market is available to partner. Families may have already exhausted SNAP and WIC monthly benefits and may not have money to purchase food at markets even if markets accept these benefits. The reach of WIC FMNP is limited. Market location and hours may not be convenient for families.

From Food Resource & Action Center. *How Pediatric Practices Are Connecting Patients to Food and Nutrition Programs: The Pros and Cons of Various Models.* American Academy of Pediatrics; 2021. Accessed March 23, 2023. https://frac.org/research/resource-library/how-pediatric-practices-are-connecting-patients-to-food-and-nutrition-programs-the-pros-and-cons-of-various-models.

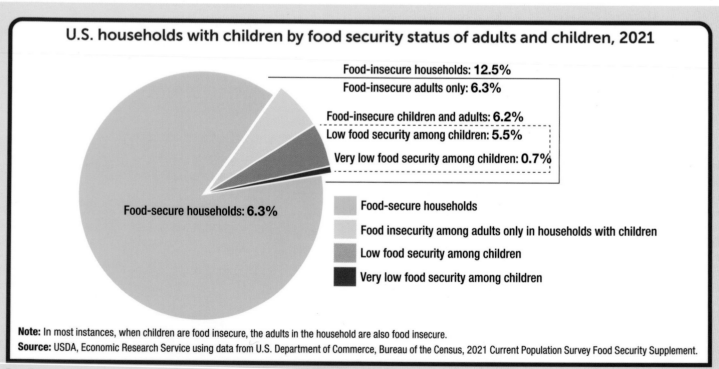

U.S. households with children by food security status of adults and children, 2021

Food-insecure households: **12.5%**

Food-insecure adults only: **6.3%**

Food-insecure children and adults: **6.2%**

Low food security among children: **5.5%**

Very low food security among children: **0.7%**

Food-secure households: **6.3%**

- Food-secure households
- Food insecurity among adults only in households with children
- Low food security among children
- Very low food security among children

Note: In most instances, when children are food insecure, the adults in the household are also food insecure.

Source: USDA, Economic Research Service using data from U.S. Department of Commerce, Bureau of the Census, 2021 Current Population Survey Food Security Supplement.

From Economic Research Service. Interactive charts and highlights. US Department of Agriculture. Accessed March 23, 2023. https://www.ers.usda.gov/topics/food-nutrition-assistance/food-security-in-the-u-s/interactive-charts-and-highlights/#childtrends.

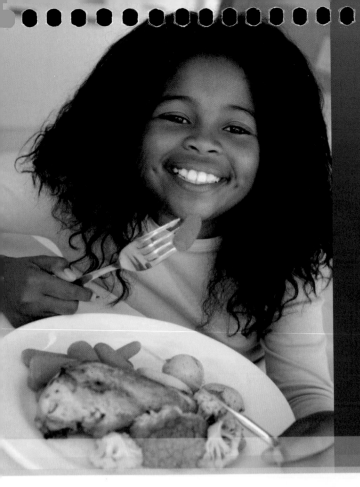

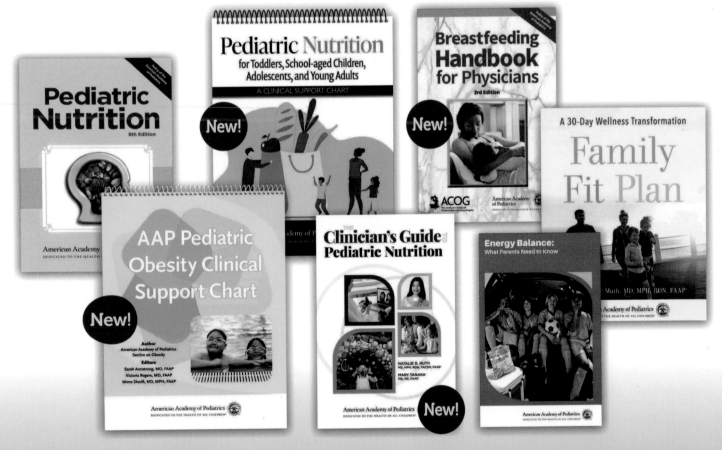

Pediatric Nutrition

for Toddlers, School-aged Children, Adolescents, and Young Adults

A CLINICAL SUPPORT CHART

AMERICAN ACADEMY OF PEDIATRICS

This point-of-care pediatric nutrition resource provides practitioners with a valuable and easy-to-use reference when evaluating and managing a pediatric patient's nutritional intake and habits. In-depth tables and charts provide specific metrics to assist the clinician, broken out by age-group, activity level, biochemical value, specific nutrient, food group, and more.

The chart can be kept on hand throughout the clinical day to support the assessment of toddlers, school-aged children, adolescents, and young adults.

Contents

For other pediatric resources, visit the
American Academy of Pediatrics at shop.aap.org.

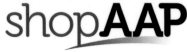

ISBN 978-1-61002-683-3

90000>

9 781610 026833

American Academy of Pediatrics

DEDICATED TO THE HEALTH OF ALL CHILDREN®